The Use of Imaging in Inflammatory Joint and Vascular Disorders

Editor

STEPHEN A. PAGET

RHEUMATIC DISEASE CLINICS OF NORTH AMERICA

www.rheumatic.theclinics.com

Consulting Editor
MICHAEL H. WEISMAN

August 2013 • Volume 39 • Number 3

ELSEVIER

1600 John F. Kennedy Boulevard • Suite 1800 • Philadelphia, Pennsylvania, 19103-2899
http://www.theclinics.com

RHEUMATIC DISEASE CLINICS OF NORTH AMERICA Volume 39, Number 3
August 2013 ISSN 0889-857X, ISBN 13: 978-1-4557-7329-9

Editor: Pamela Hetherington

Rheumatic Disease Clinics of North America (ISSN 0889-857X) is published quarterly by Elsevier Inc., 360 Park Avenue South, New York, NY 10010-1710. Months of issue are February, May, August, and November. Business and editorial offices: 1600 John F. Kennedy Boulevard, Suite 1800, Philadelphia, PA 19103-2899. Periodicals postage paid at New York, NY and additional mailing offices. Subscription prices are USD 317.00 per year for US individuals, USD 555.00 per year for US institutions, USD 156.00 per year for US students and residents, USD 374.00 per year for Canadian individuals, USD 684.00 per year for Canadian institutions, USD 444.00 per year for international individuals, USD 684.00 per year for international institutions, and USD 218.00 per year for Canadian and foreign students/residents. To receive student/resident rate, orders must be accompanied by name of affiliated institution, date of term, and the *signature* of program/residency coordinator on institution letterhead. Orders will be billed at individual rate until proof of status received. Foreign air speed delivery is included in all *Clinics* subscription prices. All prices are subject to change without notice. **POSTMASTER:** Send address changes to *Rheumatic Disease Clinics of North America,* Elsevier Health Sciences Division, Subscription Customer Service, 3251 Riverport Lane, Maryland Heights, MO 63043. **Customer Service: 1-800-654-2452 (US and Canada). From outside of the US and Canada: 314-447-8871. Fax: 314-447-8029. For print support, e-mail: JournalsCustomerService-usa@elsevier.com. For online support, e-mail: JournalsOnline Support-usa@elsevier.com.**

Reprints. For copies of 100 or more of articles in this publication, please contact the Commercial Reprints Department, Elsevier Inc., 360 Park Avenue South, New York, New York, 10010-1710; Tel.: (+1) 212-633-3813, Fax: (+1) 212-462-1935, and E-mail: reprints@elsevier.com.

Rheumatic Disease Clinics of North America is covered in *MEDLINE/PubMed (Index Medicus), Current Contents/Clinical Medicine, Science Citation Index, ISI/BIOMED,* and *EMBASE/Excerpta Medica.*

Printed and bound by CPI Group (UK) Ltd, Croydon, CR0 4YY

Transferred to digital print 2012

Contributors

CONSULTING EDITOR

MICHAEL H. WEISMAN, MD
Endowed Professor of Medicine, Director, Division of Rheumatology, Cedars-Sinai
Medical Center, Los Angeles, California

EDITOR

STEPHEN A. PAGET, MD, FACP, FACR, MACR
Physician-in-Chief Emeritus, Division of Rheumatology, Hospital For Special Surgery;
Professor of Medicine, Department of Internal Medicine, Weill Cornell Medical College,
New York, New York

AUTHORS

VIVIAN BYKERK, BSc, MD, FRCPC
Assistant Attending Physician Scientist, Hospital for Special Surgery; Associate Professor
of Medicine, Weill Cornell Medical College, New York, New York

RUSSELL CHAPIN, MD
Assistant Professor of Radiology, Department of Radiology and Radiological Science,
Medical University of South Carolina, Charleston, South Carolina

SAM R. DALVI, MD
Assistant Professor of Medicine, Division of Rheumatology and Immunology, Duke
University Medical Center, Durham, North Carolina

DAVID T. FELSON, MD, MPH
Clinical Epidemiology Research and Training Unit, Boston University School of Medicine,
Boston, Massachusetts

ALI GUERMAZI, MD, PhD
Department of Radiology, Boston University School of Medicine, Boston, Massachusetts

FAYE N. HANT, DO, MSCR
Assistant Professor of Medicine, Division of Rheumatology and Immunology, Department
of Medicine, Medical University of South Carolina, Charleston, South Carolina

DAICHI HAYASHI, MD, PhD
Department of Radiology, Boston University School of Medicine, Boston, Massachusetts

GENE G. HUNDER, MD
Professor Emeritus, Division of Rheumatology, Department of Medicine, Mayo Clinic
College of Medicine, Rochester, Minnesota

ROBERT D. INMAN, MD
Professor, Medicine and Immunology, University of Toronto; Deputy Phsycian in Chief, Research Medicine, Toronto Western Hospital, University Health Network, Toronto, Ontario, Canada

MAI MATTAR, MD
Joint Department of Medical Imaging, Mount Sinai Hospital, Women's College Hospital, University Health Network; Department of Medical Imaging, Toronto Western Hospital, Toronto, Ontario, Canada

DAVID W. MOSER, DO
Dell Children's Hospital Medical Center, Austin, Texas

HELENE PAVLOV, MD, FACR
Radiologist-in-Chief, Hospital for Special Surgery; Professor of Radiology in Orthopedic Surgery, Weill Cornell Medical College, New York, New York

NICOLÒ PIPITONE, MD, PhD
Consultant Rheumatologist, Rheumatology Unit, Department of Internal Medicine, Azienda Ospedaliera ASMN, Istituto di Ricovero e Cura a Carattere Scientifico, Reggio Emilia, Italy

FRANK W. ROEMER, MD
Department of Radiology, Boston University School of Medicine, Boston, Massachusetts

DAVID SALONEN, MD
Musculoskeletal Imaging, Department of Medical Imaging, Mount Sinai Hospital, University of Toronto, University Health Network, Toronto, Ontario, Canada

CARLO SALVARANI, MD
Head, Rheumatology Unit, Department of Internal Medicine, Azienda Ospedaliera ASMN, Istituto di Ricovero e Cura a Carattere Scientifico, Reggio Emilia, Italy

JONATHAN SAMUELS, MD
Assistant Professor of Medicine, Department of Rheumatology, New York University Langone Medical Center, New York, New York

ROBERT SCHNEIDER, MD
Attending Radiologist, Department of Radiology and Imaging, Hospital for Special Surgery; Associate Professor of Clinical Radiology, Weill Cornell Medical College, New York, New York

CAROLYN M. SOFKA, MD
Associate Professor of Radiology, Associate Attending Radiologist, Department of Radiology and Imaging, Hospital for Special Surgery, Weill Medical College of Cornell University, New York, New York

LISA C. VASANTH, MD, MSc
Assistant Attending Physician, Hospital for Special Surgery; Instructor of Medicine, Weill Cornell Medical College, New York, New York

ANNIBALE VERSARI, MD
Head, Nuclear Medicine Unit, Department of Advanced Technology, Azienda Ospedaliera ASMN, Istituto di Ricovero e Cura a Carattere Scientifico, Reggio Emilia, Italy

Contents

In large-vessel vasculitis, imaging studies are useful to document temporal artery involvement and crucial to show large-vessel involvement. Color Doppler sonography, magnetic resonance, and computed tomography show early vasculitic lesions. Angiography delineates later vascular complications well. Color Doppler sonography, magnetic resonance angiography, and computed tomography angiography can also be used to show vascular luminal changes. Positron emission tomography is very sensitive in detecting large-vessel inflammation. Imaging procedures can also be used to monitor the course of large-vessel vasculitis. In medium-vessel vasculitis, imaging studies can be used to show both vascular changes and internal organ changes.

There are many imaging methods for evaluating osteoporosis. Only a limited assessment of bone density and trabecular architecture can be done by plain radiography. Radiography is most useful in finding atraumatic fractures that are associated with osteoporosis. Radionuclide bone scanning and MRI also are useful in finding these fractures. Evaluation of bone density is most frequently assessed by dual-energy x-ray absorptiometry but can be done by other methods.

This review recounts the historical, current, and future involvement of radiology and imaging in the diagnosis, management, and follow-up of patients with various rheumatic conditions. Radiographs are the mainstay of imaging patients with rheumatic conditions, although magnetic resonance imaging and ultrasonography are routinely used for early diagnosis of disease. Computed tomography remains useful in evaluating the extent of involvement of inflammatory spondyloarthropathies that classically involve the axial skeleton and sacroiliac joints. Molecular imaging has begun to play an innovative role in evaluating patients with arthritis, aiming to identify disease earlier and provide greater specificity.

Spondyloarthropathies (SpA) are a group of disorders that primarily affect the synovial joints of the axial and appendicular skeleton of variable predilections. Plain radiography is the initial and standard method of investigation in axial SpAs. Careful evaluation of the radiographs through developing a systematic approach is indispensible in reaching the correct diagnosis. Cross-sectional imaging, in particular magnetic resonance imaging, has been increasingly used in evaluating SpAs during the early phases of the disease or when radiographic findings are equivocal. Different types of SpAs demonstrate different imaging characteristics that are important to identify to reach the correct diagnosis.

Ultrasound and Treatment Algorithms of RA and JIA   669

Sam R. Dalvi, David W. Moser, and Jonathan Samuels

Musculoskeletal ultrasound has emerged as a key tool for the diagnosis, prognosis, and management of patients with RA (rheumatoid arthritis) and other rheumatic diseases. The most important sonographic findings in RA include erosions, effusions, synovitis, and tenosynovitis. Investigators have suggested various "optimal" numbers of joints to scan in RA to assess disease activity, gauge treatment response, provide prognostic information, and guide management decisions. The complexity of pediatric sonoanatomy has delayed its validation in juvenile idiopathic arthritis, yet ultrasound reliably measures the extent of synovitis/tenosynovitis and guides precise injections.

RHEUMATIC DISEASE CLINICS
OF NORTH AMERICA

RELATED INTEREST

Orthopedic Clinics of North America, April 2013 (Volume 44, Issue 2)
Available at: http://www.orthopedic.theclinics.com/issues?
issue_key=S0030-5898(13)X0002-1
Osteoporosis and Fragility Fractures
Jason Lowe, MD, and Gary Friedlaender, MD, *Editors*

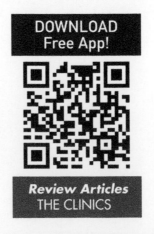

NOW AVAILABLE FOR YOUR iPhone and iPad

Foreword

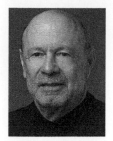

Michael H. Weisman, MD
Consulting Editor

The imaging world has collided with Rheumatology in a major way, as Dr Paget has pointed out in his series of articles in this volume. Much of the development of these modalities for rheumatic diseases has taken place as a result of work accomplished for the purpose of clinical trials outcome measurements. Now this information is being fed back directly to the care of the patient, asking questions about risk profiling for the use (or nonuse) of biologic agents or whether to intervene if the patient is not symptomatic but the disease is continuously active. In fact, these new modalities are forcing us to ask real questions about disease prevention or how to recognize "preclinical" disease in a genetically susceptible host. It is not always clear how far this will take us, but nevertheless it has moved Rheumatology forward into a role of clear intellectual engagement with not just treatment but prevention as well. Office-based ultrasound is emerging as part of the education of today's rheumatologists as much as the physical examination and the history—recognizing the need to improve on its reliability with experience and judgment is an important issue for those of us with a history of doing without it for many years. This volume is very welcome because of its timely nature and the superb job Steve Paget has done to make it clinically relevant.

Michael H. Weisman, MD
Division of Rheumatology
Cedars-Sinai Medical Center
8700 Beverly Boulevard
Los Angeles, CA 90024, USA

E-mail address:
michael.weisman@cshs.org

Rheum Dis Clin N Am 39 (2013) ix
http://dx.doi.org/10.1016/j.rdc.2013.03.006
0889-857X/13/$ – see front matter © 2013 Published by Elsevier Inc.

rheumatic.theclinics.com

Preface

The Role of Imaging Studies in Today's Rheumatology

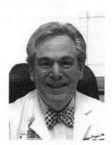

Stephen A. Paget, MD, FACP, FACR, MACR
Editor

The rheumatologist is the ultimate medical detective, using carefully collected pieces of clinical information to fill in a tapestry that defines, with clarity, the diagnosis and leads finally to a well-honed therapeutic approach to an oftentimes complex presentation. It is said that 80% of the diagnosis is based on the "clinical equation" that derives mostly from the history and an illuminating bit from the physical examination. The history and physical examination are the most powerful "biomarkers," especially in the hands of a master clinician. Although a smaller percentage of the final diagnosis is based on and guided by laboratory tests and imaging studies, these play a critically important role in further refining and clarifying the diagnosis, the extent of disease (EOD, borrowed from our oncology brethren), type, character and amount of visceral damage, and importantly, the response to treatment. The latter is key because our clinical microscope can only "see" just so far and thus we need other more sensitive tools to define with greater precision what is going on in the tissues that we are trying to protect. The perfect example of this is the fact that while we feel comfortable in defining remission and therapeutic victory in the treatment of rheumatoid arthritis with the use of validated scores such as the DAS28, a significant proportion of patients so classified have active inflammation on ultrasound and power Doppler. Stopping the development of erosions is the holy grail of the treatment of rheumatoid arthritis, one of the rheumatologist's most common foes, but while we employ all kinds of clinical proxies to augur their presence, we are in the dark without the use of imaging.

The number, sensitivity, specificity, accuracy, and diagnostic power of imaging modalities have grown exponentially over the past 30 years and with them have grown our use of and reliance on them. This has occurred because of the excellent clinical-radiologic correlations that have been made by the many rheumatologists who now have cerebral "hard drives" that contain expertise in both areas.

Rheum Dis Clin N Am 39 (2013) xi–xiv
http://dx.doi.org/10.1016/j.rdc.2013.03.001
0889-857X/13/$ – see front matter © 2013 Published by Elsevier Inc.

rheumatic.theclinics.com

The following clinical vignettes nicely highlight the role of imaging studies in the modern practice of rheumatology will also compare and contrast how decisions would have been made in the time *before* and *after* the imaging study was available.

CASE 1: RHEUMATOID ARTHRITIS

A 45-year-old woman is being treated by her rheumatologist for seropositive rheumatoid arthritis of 5 years' duration. She is at a critical point in her care because her rheumatologist believes her current regimen of low-dose prednisone, full-dose subcutaneous methotrexate, and meloxicam has not halted the inflammation or disease progression. Her rheumatologist feels that, on the basis of her clinical assessment, the persistently elevated erythrocyte sedimentation rate, C-reactive protein (CRP), and the presence of anemia and thrombocytosis, high CDAI score, and low MDHAQ, her disease is active and uncontrolled and an anti-tumor necrosis factor (TNF) should be added to her current regimen. However, she is afraid to move on to even more powerful drugs because of their potential side effects, and the devil she is comfortable with and has already learned to live with is better than the devil she doesn't know. Recent plain radiographs of the hands show no erosions or joint space narrowing, a fact that gives her comfort and supports remaining on her current regimen.

Old paradigm: The rheumatologist would base his/her recommendation on clinical grounds and plain radiographs, and the likelihood that, without a change in treatment, damage will likely ensue.

New paradigm: Given the fact that ultrasound and magnetic resonance imaging (MRI) can detect erosions 2 years *before* a plain radiograph shows them, an ultrasound of the dominant right hand was performed and the patient was able to actually see the presence of erosions, the power Doppler demonstration of active inflammation on power Doppler ("imaging sedimentation rate"), and synovial hypertrophy and tenosynovial thickening. Based on this, she agrees to starting an anti-TNF and obtaining follow-up ultrasounds at least every year to be sure that her inflammation remains tightly controlled and can be correlated with clinical parameters.

CASE 2: GIANT CELL ARTERITIS

A 82-year-old woman has recently developed severe soreness and stiffness in her shoulder and pelvic girdles, along with fatigue, headache, jaw pain with eating, and right arm pain when she raises her arm to brush her hair. Sedimentation rate is 82 mm per hour, hemoglobin 9 g%, platelets 750,000/mm^3, and CRP of 36. Right arm pulse and blood pressure are diminished when compared to the left arm. The patient is allergic to intravenous pyelogram dye; serum creatinine is 0.8.

Old paradigm: Temporal artery biopsy is performed and high-dose oral steroids are instituted.

New Paradigm: Pathophysiologic changes in the aortic wall and the superior branches of the aortic arch are challenging to diagnose and have until recently been underrecognized. To overcome such diagnostic and conceptual shortcomings that could speak to more severe disease than expected with worse short-term and long-term outcomes, a variety of noninvasive imaging techniques have been introduced in the diagnostic algorithms for functional and structural vessel changes: namely, computed tomography, MRI, aortography, duplex ultrasound, and positron emission tomography (PET) with 18-fluorodeoxyglucose (18F-FDG). However, only FDG-PET is capable of functionally and directly assessing inflammatory changes within the vessel walls. Duplex ultrasonography, computed tomography, and high-resolution MRI can demonstrate only indirect signs, such as a periluminal halo or thickening of the vessel wall. Although none of these studies are mandatory in making a decision to institute high doses of steroids in this case, the knowledge that large vessels are actively inflamed gives credence to aggressive treatment and this can be used to more accurately follow this patient's major vascular disease and its response to treatment, especially if ischemic symptoms persist. The vasculopathic phenotype of this patient's GCA can now be followed not only by the age-old erythrocyte sedimentation rate, CRP, symptoms, hemoglobin, and platelet count but disease-specific vascular monitoring.

CASE 3: ANKYLOSING SPONDYLITIS

A 33-year-old man presents to his rheumatologist for the treatment of low back pain and morning stiffness of 6 months' duration. He has no peripheral joint symptoms but he does have fatigue, anemia, elevated sedimentation rate, and weight loss of 10 pounds in 3 months. Anteroposterior radiograph of the sacroiliac joints are normal and a prior MRI of the lumbar spine showed only mild degenerative disc disease. HLA B27 is negative.

Old paradigm: A tentative diagnosis of ankylosing spondylitis is made and the patient is treated with indomethacin with only 30% improvement.

New paradigm: MRI studies of the sacroiliac joints and the spine in patients with spondyloarthritides have made a major contribution in the last decade to a better understanding of the course of the disease, early diagnosis, fulfillment of diagnostic criteria, and use as an objective outcome measure in clinical trials. Given the availability of effective anti-TNF medications and the need for as iron-clad a diagnosis as possible to warrant such expensive medications, a definitive diagnosis is mandatory and the finding of sacroiliac bone marrow edema lesions and/or erosions on MRI becomes the lynchpin of therapeutic decision-making, especially when a plain radiograph is normal.

CASE 4: OSTEONECROSIS

A 26-year-old woman with systemic lupus of 6 years' duration presents to her rheumatologist complaining of right hip pain for 1 week. She had been treated with one or another dose of prednisone throughout the course of her disease, despite the use of steroid-sparing drugs such as hydroxychloroquine and azathioprine.

Old paradigm: An anteroposterior plain radiograph of the pelvis showed no fracture, femoral head collapse, osteoporosis, or signs of infection and a total-body, 3-phase technetium bone scan showed increased uptake in the hip, an ankle, and a shoulder.

New paradigm: An MRI of the right hip is performed and shows the characteristic changes of osteonecrosis and no infection, fracture, or tumor. This is a refinement because one can define not only the pathologic bone process but also its extent and the degree of collapse.

EXPANDING THE KNOWLEDGE ABOUT PATHOPHYSIOLOGY OF JOINT DISORDERS

Ultrasound and MRI technologies have added greatly to an understanding of disease pathophysiology of rheumatoid arthritis, spondyloarthritides, and crystal-induced disorders in the characterization of bone edema lesions in rheumatoid arthritis, spondyloarthritides, and osteoarthritis and the double contour lesions and tophi in gout.

These not only have added to our basic understanding of the earliest lesions in these disorders and how they evolve with time and in the setting of treatment but also have been helpful in diagnosing disease and guiding treatment. A significant number of patients with psoriasis and no musculoskeletal symptoms are found on ultrasound and MRI to have enthesitis. The synovial enthesial complex/organ is central to the clinical and pathophysiologic understanding of spondyloarthropathies and we had no idea about its true role and anatomy prior to modern imaging.

As you read the following articles, you will be awed and impressed at how our clinical acumen and disease understanding have been expanded and made more precise with the introduction of these imaging technologies. It is likely that ultrasound will become as routine and important in our everyday activities as rheumatologists as the stethoscope and ECHO are to the cardiologist.

Stephen A. Paget, MD, FACP, FACR, MACR
Division of Rheumatology
Hospital For Special Surgery
Department of Internal Medicine
Weill Cornell Medical College
New York, New York, USA

E-mail address:
pagets@hss.edu

Imaging of Scleroderma

Russell Chapin, MD[a],*, Faye N. Hant, DO, MSCR[b]

KEYWORDS

- Scleroderma • Systemic sclerosis • Radiology • Imaging

KEY POINTS

- Systemic sclerosis is a rare autoimmune condition that can affect any organ system.
- Familiarity with skin, musculoskeletal, pulmonary, cardiac, gastrointestinal, renal, and oral imaging features in systemic sclerosis is vital for diagnosis and management of these complex patients.
- Conventional radiography, CT of the chest, echocardiography, enterography, and pan-orex dental imaging are commonly performed in patients with systemic sclerosis.
- Applications of ultrasonography and magnetic resonance imaging for musculoskeletal and cardiac evaluation in systemic sclerosis are evolving.

FEATURES OF SCLERODERMA

Systemic sclerosis (scleroderma, SSc) is a systemic connective tissue disease characterized by small-vessel vasculopathy, autoantibody production, and organ fibrosis.[1] Fibrosis in SSc can affect any organ system including the integumentary, musculoskeletal, pulmonary, cardiac, gastrointestinal (GI), and urinary systems. The classic presentation is of a 30- to 50-year-old woman with Raynaud's phenomenon (RP), skin tightening, joint and muscle pain, difficulty swallowing, and shortness of breath (**Box 1**).[2,3] SSc demonstrates a 3:1 female predilection.[4] Pulmonary involvement in the form of pulmonary arterial hypertension (PAH) and interstitial lung disease (ILD) is the major cause of mortality in SSc.[5]

Diagnostic criteria and classification schemes for SSc are debated, but include (1) localized scleroderma (morphea, linear scleroderma, mixed) and (2) systemic sclerosis. The latter includes the subsets of limited cutaneous systemic sclerosis (lcSSc, formerly known as CREST syndrome), diffuse cutaneous systemic sclerosis (dcSSC, formerly known as PSS), and systemic sclerosis sine scleroderma.[6] SSc sine scleroderma includes RP, nailfold capillaroscopy abnormalities, the presence of scleroderma autoantibodies, and visceral involvement without skin changes.[3]

[a] Department of Radiology and Radiological Science, Medical University of South Carolina, 96 Jonathan Lucas Street, Suite 210, Charleston, SC 29425, USA; [b] Department of Medicine, Division of Rheumatology and Immunology, Medical University of South Carolina, 96 Jonathan Lucas Street, Suite 912, PO Box 250637, MSC 637, Charleston, SC 29425, USA
* Corresponding author.
E-mail address: chapinrw@musc.edu

Rheum Dis Clin N Am 39 (2013) 515–546
http://dx.doi.org/10.1016/j.rdc.2013.02.017
0889-857X/13/$ – see front matter © 2013 Elsevier Inc. All rights reserved.

> **Box 1**
> **Features of systemic sclerosis**
>
> Female/male, 3:1
>
> Raynaud phenomenon
>
> Nailfold capillary changes
>
> Sclerodactyly
>
> Muscle and joint pain
>
> Dyspnea
>
> Dysphagia or reflux
>
> Limited cutaneous systemic sclerosis (lcSSc) (80%)
>
> Diffuse cutaneous systemic sclerosis (dcSSc) (20%)
>
> Disease-specific autoantibodies:
>
> • lcSSc: anticentromere and anti-Th/To antibodies
>
> • dcSSc: antitopoisomerase-1, anti-U3-RNP, and anti-RNA-polymerase III antibodies

Limited and diffuse cutaneous SSc are the predominant forms of disease, and account for the most morbidity. As many as 80% of SSc patients have lcSSc, with the 20% of patients with dcSSc demonstrating significantly greater involvement of multiple organ systems, including the lungs, heart, and GI tract.[4] The notable exception to this is the significant prevalence of PAH in lcSSc.[5,7] The presence of anticentromere antibodies (ACA) is associated with lcSSc and pulmonary hypertension (PH), and the antitopoisomerase-1 (anti–Scl-70) antibody is associated with dcSSc and ILD.[7] Anti-RNA polymerase III and anti-U3-RNP are also associated with dcSSc, whereas anti-Th/To is associated with lcSSc.[7] This article reviews the imaging features of dcSSc and lcSSc, paying particular attention to the musculoskeletal, pulmonary, and cardiac systems.

SKIN AND MUSCULOSKELETAL INVOLVEMENT IN SYSTEMIC SCLEROSIS

The hand is the most characteristic site of involvement of the skin and musculoskeletal system in SSc, and there is significant overlap in the pathophysiology of SSc in these 2 organ systems (**Box 2**). Although the typical presentation in SSc is with RP and skin tightening, patients may complain of swelling of the hands and fingers ("puffy hands")

> **Box 2**
> **Hand findings in systemic sclerosis**
>
> Acral soft-tissue thinning
>
> Digital pitting and ulcerations
>
> Acroosteolysis
>
> Acral and periarticular soft-tissue calcification
>
> Flexion contractures
>
> Mild degenerative or erosive joint findings
>
> Tendon friction rubs

and joint pain, mimicking rheumatoid arthritis (RA).[8] Articular symptoms are reported in approximately 10% to 60% of scleroderma patients at the time of diagnosis, and are frequently the initial manifestation of disease.[8] Typical manifestations of SSc in the hands include RP, digital skin thickening (sclerodactyly), acral soft-tissue thinning, digital pitting and ulcerations, acroosteolysis, calcinosis, tendon friction rubs, flexion contractures, and arthralgias.

RP is exacerbated by emotional stress or cold, and consists of white (pallor) to blue (cyanosis) to red (reperfusion) finger discoloration corresponding to vasospasm, ischemia, and reactive hyperemia, respectively.[9] RP is reported in 95% of SSc patients.[2] Though typical of SSc, RP can be seen in isolation (primary RP) or be associated with other vasculitides and collagen vascular diseases (secondary RP), or chemical, drug, or environmental exposures.[9]

The skin is the most commonly involved organ in SSc.[10] Skin thickening and induration typically occur in the hands and face. Telangiectasias are also frequently seen. Patients with lcSSc have skin involvement distal to the elbows and knees, whereas patients with dcSSc have truncal and more proximal limb involvement. The extent of skin disease is assessed and monitored using the modified Rodnan skin score (mRSS), which is based on clinical evaluation of skin thickness at 17 sites.[11] High-frequency ultrasonography offers potential as an objective measure of skin involvement and a method for discriminating edematous from fibrotic changes, but has demonstrated poor interobserver and intraobserver reproducibility.[12] Magnetic resonance imaging (MRI) can also demonstrate abnormalities of the skin and subcutaneous tissues (**Fig. 1**). One study of 18 patients with SSc and musculoskeletal symptoms evaluated by whole-body MRI showed subcutaneous and fascial thickening and enhancement in 89%.[13] Of note, these findings did not correlate with the mRSS. MRI and ultrasonography are also capable of delineating localized scleroderma (morphea) and excluding underlying myositis (**Fig. 2**).

Acral changes in SSc include RP, sclerodactyly, soft-tissue thinning, digital pits and ulcers, and acroosteolysis (**Fig. 3**). The shared pathogenesis of these lesions is likely

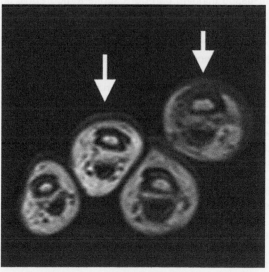

Fig. 1. T1 axial MR image of the second to fourth fingers demonstrates thickened low signal of the dorsal skin (*arrows*) consistent with scleroderma.

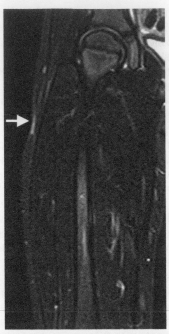

Fig. 2. Coronal short-tau inversion recovery MR image of the right thigh shows focal subcutaneous increased signal (*arrow*) in a 4-year-old with morphea.

endothelial dysfunction with upregulation of vasoconstrictors and downregulation of vasodilators.[14] Acral soft-tissue thinning is strongly associated with RP and is reported in 15% to 80% of patients with SSc.[8] There is an association between digital ulcers and acroosteolysis, suggesting a shared pathogenesis of vascular injury and vasospasm.[15] Acral soft-tissue thinning can be a subtle radiographic finding, and can be assessed by comparing the depth of the soft tissue from the tip of the distal phalanx to the skin surface with the width of the base of the distal phalanx. A ratio of less than 0.2 is consistent with acral soft-tissue thinning (**Fig. 4**A).[16]

The reported frequency of acroosteolysis in SSc is also highly variable, ranging from 20% to 80%.[8,15] Acroosteolysis is usually accompanied by acral soft-tissue thinning (see **Fig. 4**B), but the degree of bone resorption may be disproportionate.[17] Acroosteolysis tends to involve the palmar surface initially, and can progress to the appearance of a pencil tip (**Fig. 5**).[8] Bone resorption may also be seen at the superior margin of the medial aspect of ribs 2 to 6, the distal radius and ulna, the distal clavicle, and the angle of the mandible.[17]

Soft-tissue calcifications are noted in the hands in 10% to 30% of patients and may be subcutaneous or periarticular, with a predilection for the fingertips (**Fig. 6**).[8] These calcifications are likely caused by local vascular and fibrotic changes. Periarticular calcifications may also be seen beyond the hands and can have a "sheet-like" or lobular appearance (**Fig. 7**). Asymmetric distribution in the dominant hand and involvement over bony prominences, such as the fingertips, elbows, and knees, suggest that focal injury may play a role (**Fig. 8**).[8] Some investigators have shown an association between calcinosis and lcSSC, and periarticular calcifications have been proposed as a cause of joint erosions in SSc.[15,18] Paraspinal calcifications can also be seen and can lead to narrowing of the spinal canal.[19]

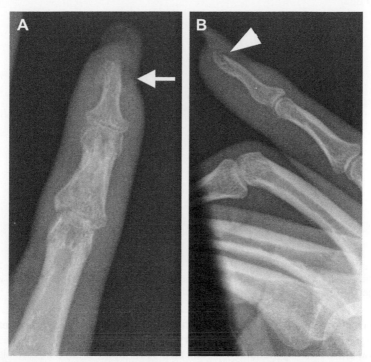

Fig. 3. Frontal (*A*) and lateral (*B*) radiographs of the fifth digit in a patient with SSc. There is focal skin ulceration (*arrow*) at the dorsal lateral aspect of the fifth finger. There is underlying focal bone erosion (*arrowhead*). Digital ulcers may be seen in systemic sclerosis (SSc), and this patient was diagnosed with dry gangrene.

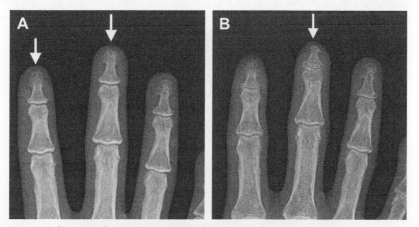

Fig. 4. Frontal-finger radiographs in 2008 (*A*) and 2012 (*B*) demonstrate the progression of acral soft-tissue thinning and mild osteolysis of the distal phalanx of the third digit in this patient with scleroderma. In 2008 (*A*), there is subtle thinning of the soft tissue of the second and third finger tufts (*arrows*); this is appreciated in comparison with the width of the distal phalanx and the adjacent fourth finger tuft. In 2012 (*B*), there is progressive thinning of the soft tissue of the third finger tuft with a more tapered appearance of the soft tissue and bone of the distal phalanx, consistent with mild acroosteolysis (*arrow*).

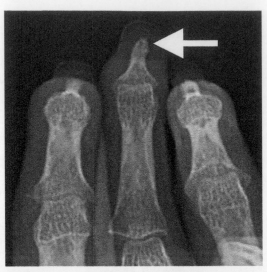

Fig. 5. There is significant acroosteolysis of the second, third, and fourth fingers, with the third finger tuft having the appearance of a sharpened pencil (*arrow*).

Tendon friction rubs (TFR) are a classic physical-examination finding in patients with SSc, and present as palpable crepitus over the tendon sheaths of the wrists, fingers, knees, and ankles during motion.[8] TFR can also occur at the shoulders and elbows of patients with SSc. TFR are present in 53% of patients with dcSSc but in only 5% of lcSSc patients.[20] The presence of tendon friction rubs is strongly correlated with pulmonary fibrosis and morbidity. TFR are present early in the disease, sometimes before skin changes.[21,22] Given this fact, early recognition of TFR is significant. Based on pathologic findings, TFR are likely secondary to fibrous thickening of the tendon sheaths.[22] On ultrasonography, the thickness of the A2 finger pulley has been shown to be significantly

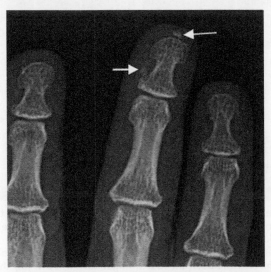

Fig. 6. There are small foci of soft-tissue calcification at the tip and radial aspect of the third finger (*arrows*). This location is typical of calcification in SSc.

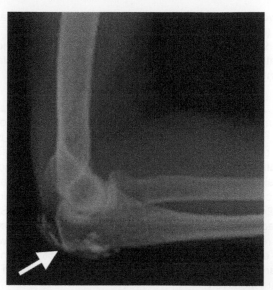

Fig. 7. Lateral elbow radiograph demonstrates soft-tissue calcification dorsal to the olecranon (*arrow*). Soft-tissue calcifications frequently occur at pressure sites such as the dorsal elbow.

greater in SSc patients than in controls.[23] Soft-tissue thickening surrounding the ankle tendons has been noted on MRI, and significant tendon abnormalities have been seen with both MRI and ultrasonography in the absence of clinical findings.[21]

Flexion contractures of the hands are typical and are observed in approximately 30% of patients with SSc. This condition has been described as a periarticular fibrotic

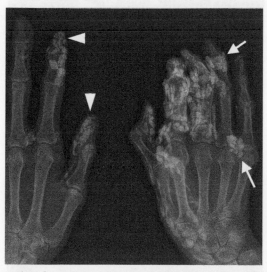

Fig. 8. Hand radiographs of a patient with chronic SSc demonstrate diffuse cutaneous and periarticular calcifications (*arrows*), which have a lobular or cloud-like appearance. Calcifications are more extensive distally (*arrowheads*) and greater in the right hand. Osteopenia is noted, and may be secondary to disuse because of the calcifications and joint contractures.

pattern of joint involvement.[18,24] Flexion contractures are most apparent at the metacarpophalangeal (MCP) and interphalangeal (IP) joints on physical examination and radiography (**Fig. 9**). These contractures are secondary to skin, synovial, or capsular fibrosis in SSc patients.[15,24] Flexion contractures have been associated with dcSSc, the anti–Scl-70 antibody, and pulmonary fibrosis.[18]

Arthritis

Joint complaints are common in SSc, and are generally ascribed to arthralgia rather than true arthritis.[22] However, focal joint-space findings of arthritis, including narrowing, periarticular osteopenia, and erosions, are frequently reported in hand radiographs of SSc patients.[15,18,24–26] In particular, erosions are reported in up to 40% of patients.[26] Several studies have assessed the presence of these imaging characteristics. Blocka and colleagues[25] found joint-space narrowing, periarticular osteopenia, and erosions in 24%, 9%, and 27% of patients with advanced SSc, respectively. Baron and colleagues[26] reported these same findings with a frequency of 34%, 42%, and 40%, respectively. In another study, joint-space narrowing, periarticular osteopenia, and erosions were seen 54%, 13%, and 5% of hand radiographs.[24] Finally, Avouac and colleagues[15] reported these same findings in 28%, 23%, and 21% of patients, respectively.

Although overlap with RA is present in approximately 5% of SSc patients, the appearance of erosions in these series is distinct from RA.[27,28] Evaluation for anticyclic citrullinated peptide antibodies (anti-CCP) is helpful when RA-SSc overlap is suspected.

The distribution of erosions in SSc is different from that of RA. Most commonly, bone erosions in SSc are noted at the MCP joints, particularly the dorsal aspect, and the distal interphalangeal (DIP) joints, where they may mimic psoriatic and

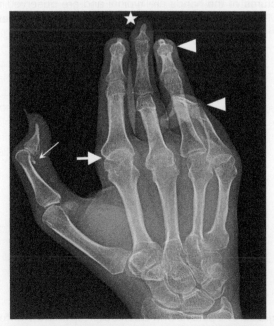

Fig. 9. Hand radiograph demonstrates metacarpophalangeal (MCP) joint (*arrow*) and interphalangeal (IP) joint (*arrowheads*) flexion contractures, with periarticular soft-tissue calcification of the thumb (*thin arrow*) and acroosteolysis of the third distal phalanx (*star*).

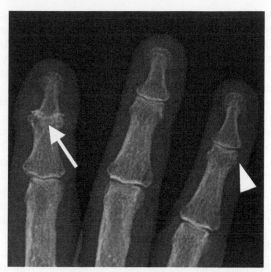

Fig. 10. Finger radiographs of a patient with scleroderma show joint-space narrowing of the second distal interphalangeal (DIP) joint with central erosion (*arrow*) in a pattern similar to that of erosive osteoarthritis. A very small marginal erosion is present at the fourth DIP joint (*arrowhead*).

particularly erosive osteoarthritis (**Fig. 10**).[18,24,25] A distinctive carpometacarpal (CMC) erosion with associated radial subluxation has been reported (**Fig. 11**).[8] Several theories have been proposed for these erosions, the most likely of which, supported by synovial biopsy results, is that patients with SSc exhibit a milder form of synovitis that chronically takes the form of synovial fibrosis rather than pannus formation.[25] The erosions of SSc have been described as small, discrete, and less invasive than

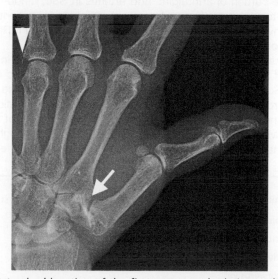

Fig. 11. There is lateral subluxation of the first metacarpal relative to the trapezium with erosion (*arrow*) of the trapezium. A small fourth-digit periarticular calcification is noted (*arrowhead*).

those of RA.[26] Erosions in SSc could be caused by pressure from joint contractures and subluxation, and this correlates with the reported frequency of erosions involving the MCP joints.[25] Osteolysis is noted at nonsynovial sites in SSc including the forearm and ribs, and it has been postulated that hand erosions are merely an extension of this.[25] Finally, the erosions could be related to juxta-articular calcifications, which are frequently seen in SSc.[15]

The predominant findings of hand arthrosis in SSc can be classified by the following types: (1) minimal change, (2) periarticular fibrotic, (3) degenerative, or (4) inflammatory.[18,24] La Montagna and colleagues[24] were able to uniquely categorize 75 of 76 patients based on these groups, and found a prevalence of 30%, 13%, and 13% for types 2, 3, and 4, respectively. Erre and colleagues[18] found a pattern of minimal change in 20%, periarticular fibrosis in 34%, distal degeneration in 22%, and erosive disease in 20% of patients. Based on these results, this group described the degenerative pattern (type 3) in SSc as an "arthropathy unrelated to the disease." Of these types, periarticular fibrotic arthrosis is the most characteristic of SSc (**Box 3**).

Musculoskeletal Ultrasonography and MRI

Relatively few studies have examined the role of ultrasonography and MRI in the characterization of SSc joint disease. Using ultrasonography, Cuomo and colleagues[29] found synovial proliferation (which may be fibrotic or inflamed), increased synovial Doppler flow, and erosions in 42%, 24%, and 11% of SSc patients, respectively. Another study reported erosions in 53% and synovitis in 20% of patients with SSc studied by ultrasonography.[30] On hand MRI, Low and colleagues[31] reported a high prevalence of inflammatory findings including synovitis (47%), tenosynovitis (47%), erosions (41%), and bone edema (53%) in 17 symptomatic patients (**Fig. 12**). These MRI findings did not correlate with clinical evidence of synovitis and did not show any apparent association with anti-CCP to suggest overlap with RA. A possible explanation for synovial and tenosynovial fluid in SSc is that it occurs secondary to flexion and subluxation of the joints, in addition to tendon compression by peritendinous fibrosis. Given the burden of arthralgias and arthritis in SSc, randomized controlled trials are needed to evaluate effective treatment regimens for patients with SSc and associated joint involvement. In such trials, ultrasonography and MRI may be helpful for patient selection and evaluation of treatment response.

Although often underappreciated, muscle involvement is reported in more than 70% of SSc patients.[19] Similar to the distinction between arthralgias and arthritis, muscle involvement in SSc has been termed myopathy or myositis, with the former demonstrating bland fibrous tissue and the latter showing true inflammation.[19] Weakness or myalgia involving the hip girdle is the most common symptom of muscle involvement in SSc. On MRI, myositis is characterized by intramuscular high T2 signal consistent with edema.[22] Areas of muscular high signal can be targeted for biopsy as

---

Box 3
Arthritis in systemic sclerosis

Type 1: Minimal joint change

Type 2: Flexion contracture

Type 3: Degenerative

Type 4: Inflammatory/erosive[a]

  [a] If present, erosions are usually at the MCP, DIP, or first CMC joint.

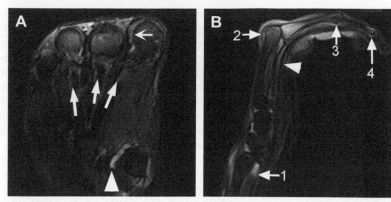

Fig. 12. T2 fat-saturated images of the right hand in the coronal (*A*) and sagittal (*B*) plane demonstrate flexion contractures typical of scleroderma, which make MRI challenging. Saturation of the subcutaneous and intraosseous fat signal is incomplete. In *A*, there is fluid signal surrounding the flexor tendons of the second to fourth digits (*arrows*), and fluid signal of the thumb carpal-metacarpal joint (*arrowhead*) as well as the second MCP joint (*thin arrow*). On the sagittal image (*B*), there is increased fluid in the distal radial ulnar (1) and in the MCP (2), proximal interphalangeal (3), and DIP (4) joints of the fourth finger. Subtle fluid is seen along the fourth flexor tendon (*arrowhead*). Rheumatoid factors were negative in this patient.

necessary. Chronically, areas of high T1 MRI signal indicate muscle atrophy. Involvement is typically symmetric involving the hip adductors, abductors, and quadriceps, and the appearance is identical to that of dermatomyositis, but distinct from eosinophilic fasciitis (**Fig. 13**).[22] One MRI study of 18 patients with SSc and musculoskeletal symptoms found muscle edema signal suggestive of myositis in 78%, fascial abnormalities in 89%, and subcutaneous infiltration in 89%.[13] Of interest, the presence of myositis in SSc has been correlated with myocardial disease.[22]

PULMONARY INVOLVEMENT IN SYSTEMIC SCLEROSIS
Interstitial Lung Disease

SSc-related ILD (SSc-ILD) is the most common pulmonary manifestation of SSc and, along with PH, is the leading cause of death in SSc.[4] Patients with SSc-ILD can

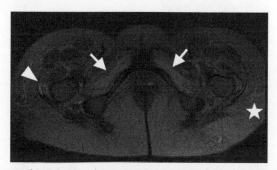

Fig. 13. T2 fat-saturated MR image demonstrates increased signal in the bilateral adductor brevis and obturator externus muscles (*arrows*), consistent with myositis. There is also milder signal abnormality deep to the iliotibial band (*arrowhead*) and in the subcutaneous fat (*star*) bilaterally.

present in many ways, so clinicians must remain observant in screening and monitoring patients. Clinically, patients can range from asymptomatic to having dyspnea on exertion (DOE), nonproductive cough, atypical chest pain, and fatigue. Physical examination may be normal; however, the most common finding in SSc-ILD is fine, inspiratory "Velcro-like" crackles at the lung bases. Any patient with SSc can develop SSc-ILD, including patients with dcSSc, lcSSc, SSc sine scleroderma, and those with overlap syndromes. On high-resolution computed tomography (HRCT), two-thirds of SSc patients show evidence of SSc-ILD while 30% to 40% of SSc patients have significant pulmonary symptoms.[4,10,32] Chest HRCT is necessary for detecting, accurately characterizing, and appropriately treating lung disease in SSc.

Traditionally, SSc-ILD was equated to idiopathic pulmonary fibrosis, which is described as usual interstitial pneumonia (UIP) at pathology and HRCT. It is now accepted that most SSc-ILD has the imaging and histopathologic pattern of nonspecific interstitial pneumonia (NSIP).[33,34] On HRCT, both NSIP and UIP demonstrate reticular interstitial markings predominantly involving the posterior basilar aspects of the lower lobes. Traction bronchiectasis is seen in both UIP and NSIP, but more extensively in the former.[35] NSIP is best characterized by ground-glass opacities (**Fig. 14**), whereas UIP is characterized by the appearance of a "honeycomb" of small homogenously sized grouped or stacked cyst-like lucencies that often reach the pleura (**Fig. 15**).[36,37] NSIP commonly demonstrates subpleural sparing (**Fig. 16**).[36] Honeycombing can still be seen in 20% to 30% of NSIP, and ground-glass opacity is often present in UIP.[4,36] Despite this overlap, the positive predictive value of computed tomography (CT) is 80% to 90% for UIP and approximately 50% for NSIP.[36] Other pulmonary diseases that may also occur in patients with SSc and should be differentiated from NSIP include hypersensitivity pneumonitis, drug reactions, pulmonary hemorrhage, malignancy, pneumoconiosis, and aspiration pneumonia.

The accuracy of conventional radiography for detecting and characterizing lung disease in SSc is significantly limited. HRCT is more sensitive than radiography at detecting early ILD, and can better quantify the degree of interstitial fibrosis. In a small group of SSc patients with an ILD prevalence of 91% at HRCT, only 39% showed convincing radiographic evidence for ILD.[38] With radiography, there is overlap in the appearance of NSIP and UIP, with only faint bibasilar reticular abnormalities

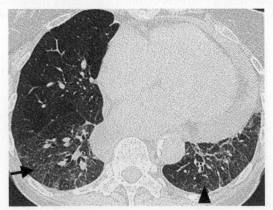

Fig. 14. Chest computed tomography (CT) shows peripheral basilar predominant ground-glass opacity (*arrowhead*) and fine interstitial lines (*arrow*), typical of nonspecific interstitial pneumonia (NSIP).

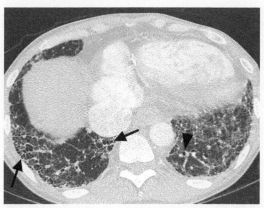

Fig. 15. Chest CT shows increased interstitial marking at the lung bases with a peripheral predominance. There is traction bronchiectasis (*arrowhead*), and there are stacked cysts at the far periphery of the lung with a honeycomb appearance (*arrows*). Honeycomb areas can be seen in SSc, and the appearance in this case is consistent with usual interstitial pneumonia (UIP).

visible early in the disease (**Fig. 17**), and thicker peripheral interstitial opacities accompanied by traction bronchiectasis and volume loss with more advanced disease (**Fig. 18**).

Pulmonary assessment in SSc requires pulmonary function testing (PFT), 6-minute walk testing, and HRCT. Abnormal HRCT findings correlate with reductions in forced expiratory volume (FEV), forced vital capacity (FVC), total lung capacity (TLC), and diffusion capacity (DLCO).[5] However, HRCT abnormalities can be seen when PFTs are normal, and PFT findings may reveal disease in patients with a normal HRCT.[5] It is therefore recommended that all patients with SSc undergo baseline HRCT and PFT screening with spirometry and diffusion.[4] Patients with SSc-ILD have restrictive pulmonary physiology, and decreases in FVC, FEV, and DLCO at PFT are generally proportional. A disproportionate decrease in DLCO relative to FEV and FVC may be seen in SSc-ILD, but should raise suspicion for PAH.[5]

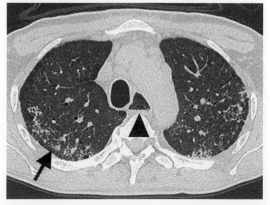

Fig. 16. Chest CT in another patient shows peripheral interstitial thickening in the superior lungs (*arrowhead*) with sparing of the most peripheral lung (*arrow*), typical of NSIP.

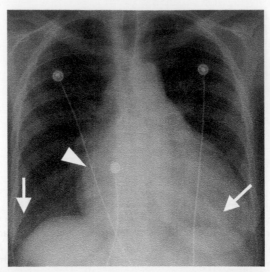

Fig. 17. Chest radiograph in a patient with SSc demonstrates ill-defined increased interstitial markings at the lung bases (*arrows*). This patient is the same shown on CT in **Fig. 15** with a significant UIP pattern. Also, there is right atrial enlargement (*arrowhead*), which can be seen secondary to pulmonary hypertension or diastolic dysfunction.

The presence or absence of HRCT findings in SSc correlates with differences in treatment response and mortality. Patients with no HRCT lung disease on initial evaluation are less likely to develop symptoms or HRCT evidence of SSc-ILD in follow-up.[39] In the scleroderma lung study, the presence of fibrotic SSc-ILD correlated with a greater treatment effect of cyclophosphamide.[40] In another study, patients with HRCT abnormalities involving more than 20% of the lungs had a significantly more rapid progression of lung disease and greater mortality than patients with less

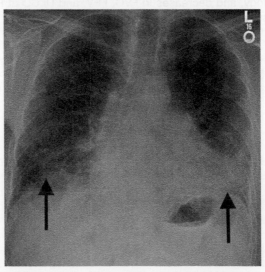

Fig. 18. Chest radiograph in a patient with advanced interstitial lung disease and pulmonary fibrosis shows coarse interstitial markings at the lung bases (*arrows*) and volume loss.

extensive findings on CT.[41] Compared with other connective tissue disease–related ILD, there is evidence that the presence of a UIP pattern in SSc-ILD does not predict a worse outcome than an NSIP pattern.[42] This finding suggests that the use of a visual scoring system based on the volume of lung involvement (eg, 0%–25%, 26%–50%, 51%–75%, 76%–100%) may be more useful.[4]

In most ILDs, areas of ground-glass pulmonary attenuation on HRCT are suggestive of cellular infiltration and the potential for treatment response. Although there is an in-flammatory component in SSc-ILD, there is some evidence that ground glass on CT in SSc-ILD may not be cellular, reversible, or predictive of a treatment response.[4,5,43]

Other Pulmonary Manifestations

In patients with SSc, pulmonary and pleural diseases other than NSIP are as common, and likely more so, as in the general population. Peripheral reticular opacities and sub-tle changes in attenuation mimicking mild NSIP are frequently seen in the dependent portion of the lung secondary to atelectasis and perfusion changes alone. For this reason, a portion of the HRCT examination should be performed with prone posi-tioning. The presence of significantly asymmetric or unilateral middle or upper lobe consolidation or ground-glass opacity is consistent with infectious pneumonia, partic-ularly in patients who are immunocompromised because of steroid and/or other immunosuppressive therapies. Cryptogenic organizing pneumonia (COP) has been reported in SSc and can also demonstrate areas of ground glass, but more typically demonstrates patchy peribronchovascular and subpleural consolidation and nodular-ity.[10,44] Drug toxicity may be seen in SSc, and can have the appearance of diffuse ground glass or a COP or NSIP pattern.[10,45]

Cardiogenic edema may develop secondary to left ventricular diastolic dysfunction in SSc, and should have a distinct appearance of basilar predominant ground glass with peribronchovascular, fissural, and peripheral interlobular septal thickening and effusions. In the absence of heart failure, pleural effusions may be seen in 7% of SSc patients.[46] Extrinsic compromise of pulmonary function secondary to myopathy is also common in SSc.[5] This condition is best characterized by clinical examination and PFT, but may demonstrate hypoventilatory changes such as atelectasis at CT.

Esophageal dysmotility is common in SSc and may lead to aspiration. Esophageal dysmotility has been proposed as a contributing factor in SSc-ILD. A correlation be-tween dysmotility and SSc-ILD has been noted in several studies but not in others.[5] The proposed pathogenesis of this association is occult aspiration. On chest CT or radiographs, significant acute aspiration most typically shows perihilar multifocal opacities in the posterior segments of the upper lobes and superior segments of the lower lobes.[47]

Several population studies have shown a significant increased risk of lung cancer in SSc, but have been contradicted by another study showing no increased risk.[5] Pro-posed mechanisms of lung cancer in SSc include chronic lung injury and repair as well as chronic cyclophosphamide administration. Although this association warrants further study, the appearance of an enlarging focal nodule or spiculated mass on chest CT is most characteristic of a bronchogenic cancer. On the other hand, mild medias-tinal lymph node enlargement in the presence of an NSIP pattern typical of SSc-ILD should not significantly increase suspicion for neoplasm, as nodal enlargement has been reported in 60% of patients with NSIP.[4]

Pulmonary Hypertension

PH is defined as a mean pulmonary arterial pressure of 25 mm Hg and greater, or peak systolic pulmonary arterial pressure of at least 35 mm Hg at rest. In SSc, PH may be secondary to ILD or cardiomyopathy with diastolic dysfunction, or can occur as a primary event, in which case it is best termed pulmonary arterial hypertension (PAH).[48] In one cohort, 23% of SSc patients had findings of ILD without PH, 20% had PH without ILD (PAH), and 18% had both.[49] Overall, 10% to 15% of SSc patients have PAH, which is a leading cause of death in patients with SSc.[48] There is a significant association between lcSSc and PAH, with two-thirds of SSc patients with PAH having lcSSc.[48] For this reason, patients with lcSSc may be screened more frequently for PH; however, annual screening for PH with echocardiography should occur regardless of SSc subtype (lcSSc, dcSSc, SSc sine scleroderma, or overlap).

Imaging of Pulmonary Hypertension

The gold standard for the detection of PH is right heart catheterization, but Doppler echocardiography (DE) is a noninvasive, accurate, and efficient method to screen for PH. Compared with right heart catheterization DE can overestimate or underestimate pulmonary arterial pressure, but has an approximate sensitivity and specificity of 90% and 75%, respectively.[50] Measurement of the peak regurgitant velocity across the tricuspid valve with DE allows for calculation of the peak systolic pressure difference between the right atrium and right ventricle.[50] The right atrial pressure is usually estimated to be 5 mm Hg, so the peak systolic right ventricular pressure, corresponding to the peak pulmonary arterial pressure, can be calculated (**Fig. 19**). When significant changes or abnormalities consistent with PH are detected at Doppler screening, right heart catheterization is performed.

CT features that indicate PH are useful, despite chest CT being most commonly performed for evaluation of scleroderma lung disease rather than PH (**Box 4**). One exception to this is CT pulmonary angiography performed to evaluate for chronic thromboembolic disease. Chronic pulmonary thromboembolism is not significantly more common in SSc than in the general population, but CT pulmonary angiography may be requested in SSc patients with declining respiratory function. In addition to enlargement of the main pulmonary arteries, vascular findings of chronic thromboembolic disease include eccentric thrombi, webs, irregular narrowings, obstruction, tortuosity, and calcification of the peripheral pulmonary arteries.[51] In the pulmonary parenchyma, scars and a mosaic appearance caused by patchy low attenuation of

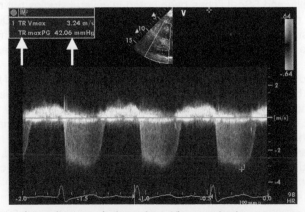

Fig. 19. Doppler echocardiogram during tricuspid regurgitation measures velocity at the tricuspid valve from which the pressure gradient from the right atrium to ventricle is calculated (*arrows*). In this patient with pulmonary hypertension at rest, the gradient is 42 mm Hg, which corresponds to a peak systolic right ventricular/arterial pressure of 47 mm Hg.

Box 4
Chest CT findings in systemic sclerosis
NSIP > UIP pattern of interstitial lung disease
Pulmonary Hypertension
• Large main pulmonary artery
• Right heart enlargement
• Mosaic lung attenuation
Dilated esophagus
Pleural or pericardial effusions
Pneumonia, congestive heart failure, bronchogenic cancer

underperfused areas may be present. Mosaic attenuation may be seen in primary arterial (PAH) or post-thrombotic PH, and demonstrates less air trapping on expiratory CT than similar-appearing areas in cases of small airways disease.[52]

Most CT findings of PH are a reflection of elevated pulmonary arterial, right ventricular, and right atrial pressure with reflux across the tricuspid valve. These findings include pulmonary arterial enlargement, right ventricular hypertrophy, right ventricular and right atrial enlargement, reflux of contrast into the inferior vena cava (IVC), and bronchial arterial enlargement (**Fig. 20**).[53,54] Cardiac changes on CT secondary to PH usually become apparent in long-standing significant PH, and are therefore specific but not sensitive. Reflux of contrast into the IVC depends on the rate of contrast injection during CT. At high contrast injection rates used for CT pulmonary angiography, reflux of contrast into the IVC has a sensitivity of 81% and specificity of 69% for PAH and right heart disease (**Fig. 21**).[54]

Enlargement of the main pulmonary artery may be an earlier finding in SSc patients with PH of any cause. In patients with lung disease, a main pulmonary arterial diameter of 29 mm or more has a reported sensitivity of 84% and a specificity of 75% for PH.[55] In another study of patients with a variety of underlying chest diseases, a ratio of main pulmonary arterial to ascending aortic diameter of greater than 1 was 70% sensitive

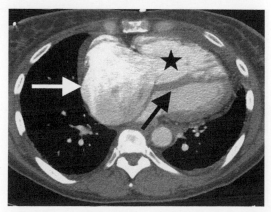

Fig. 20. CT of the chest with contrast demonstrates enlargement of the right atrium (*white arrow*) and right ventricle (*star*), with flattening and displacement of the interventricular septum toward the left ventricle (*black arrow*).

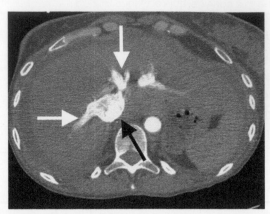

Fig. 21. Chest CT with contrast during the arterial phase in another patient with SSc and pulmonary hypertension demonstrates reflux of contrast into the inferior vena cava (*black arrow*) and hepatic veins (*white arrows*) from the right atrium, consistent with pulmonary hypertension and diastolic dysfunction.

and 92% specific for predicting PH (**Fig. 22**).[56] However, a larger and more detailed study found that the correlation between pulmonary arterial enlargement and PH is present, but not as strongly as in patients with ILD.[57] A threshold main pulmonary arterial diameter of 25 mm resulted in a sensitivity and specificity for PH of 86% and 41%, respectively, in patients with ILD. However, in patients without ILD a significantly different cutoff value of 32 mm was necessary to obtain a sensitivity and specificity of 47% and 93%, respectively. Corroborating the findings of other investigators, there was also little correlation between PH and ILD in this study.[57]

Cardiac MRI is the accepted standard for evaluation of cardiac structure, function, and viability, particularly of the right atrium and ventricle.[58,59] However, comparison of cardiac MRI with right heart catheterization for evaluation of PH has yielded mixed results.[60] The amount of leftward interventricular septal curvature on MRI has been correlated with pulmonary arterial pressure (**Fig. 23**) and has demonstrated responsiveness to vasodilator treatment, but these results were obtained in patients with

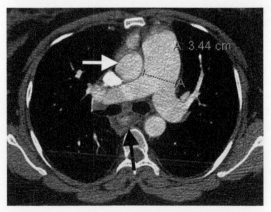

Fig. 22. CT of the chest with contrast in a patient with SSc shows that the pulmonary arterial diameter is measured as 3.4 cm, and is greater than that of the adjacent ascending aorta (*white arrow*). The esophagus is distended and filled with debris (*black arrow*).

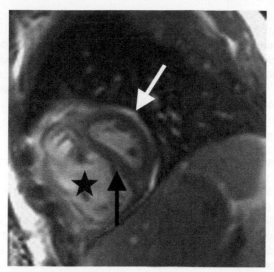

Fig. 23. Short-axis MR image of the heart shows flattening and subtle bowing of the inter-ventricular septum (*black arrow*) away from the right ventricle (*star*) and toward the left ventricle (*white arrow*), creating a D-shaped left ventricle.

advanced PH.[61] One intriguing finding with cardiac MRI is that patients with PH demonstrate delayed contrast enhancement at the junction of the right ventricular walls with the septum (**Fig. 24**). This characteristic has been shown in several studies in 23 of 25, 15 of 15, and 13 of 20 patients.[62–64] However, these studies were also per-formed in patients with severe PH, and no correlation was found between the degree of enhancement and the severity of PH. Delayed enhancement on MRI corresponds to

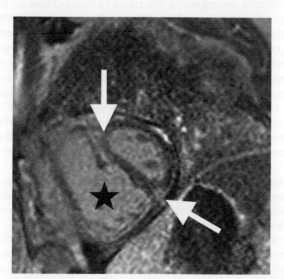

Fig. 24. Delayed postcontrast short-axis cardiac MR image demonstrates enhancement (*arrows*) where the superior and inferior walls of the right ventricle (*star*) meet the septum. This finding is described in pulmonary hypertension.

fibrosis and is thought to occur at the right ventricular-septal junction because of increased stress at this location.[63]

Treatment options for PH include calcium-channel blockers, prostacyclin analogues, phosphodiesterase inhibitors, and endothelin antagonists.[5] When present, vasoreactivity during right heart catheterization may justify the use of calcium-channel blockers.[5] Treatment of PH in SSc is significantly complicated by the frequent coexistence of diastolic dysfunction and ILD.

CARDIAC INVOLVEMENT IN SYSTEMIC SCLEROSIS

The most significant cardiac complication of SSc is right-sided heart failure (cor pulmonale) secondary to PH. However, primary cardiac involvement in SSc is common. At autopsy, up to 80% of SSc patients are reported to have myocardial fibrosis.[65] Clinical symptoms of cardiac disease are reported in 15% to 35% of patients.[66] Cardiac involvement in SSc has a poor prognosis, with 70% mortality at 5 years.[67] Approximately 20% of mortality from SSc can be attributed to cardiac disease independent of PH.[66] Myocardial fibrosis and coronary microvascular disease are the disorders underlying most primary cardiac disease in SSc, and can lead to diastolic or systolic dysfunction and arrhythmias.

Myocardial Disease

Myocardial fibrosis is the signature cardiac disease of SSc and may manifest as heart failure, diastolic dysfunction, or arrhythmia.[67] Imaging findings of cardiac fibrosis on radiographs, CT, and DE rely on indirect and variable signs that are primarily related to restricted ventricular filling and secondary enlargement (see **Fig. 17**).[68] Catheter-directed myocardial biopsy is invasive and is subject to sampling error.[65] Cardiac MRI excels at detecting myocardial fibrosis, which appears as delayed enhancement in a noncoronary distribution on postcontrast images. A recent MRI study by Tzelepis and colleagues[65] found evidence of fibrosis in 66% of SSc patients. Delayed contrast enhancement in SSc is described in the basal to mid-portion of the left ventricle, involving the septum and free wall, and has a linear and spiculated appearance (**Fig. 25**).[65] Cardiac fibrosis in SSc also demonstrates subendocardial sparing. Of note, the degree of fibrosis estimated by imaging in this study was positively associated with arrhythmias.[65]

Low-grade myocardial inflammation has been detected in SSc biopsy samples, and may be related to fibrosis.[67] However, the appearance of myocarditis on MRI should be distinguished from fibrosis, based on the finding of subepicardial involvement and increased signal on T2 in myocarditis and not in fibrosis.[65] Myocarditis has been associated with skeletal myositis.[67,69] One series of patients with SSc and musculoskeletal symptoms demonstrated MRI findings consistent with skeletal myositis in 78% of patients.[13]

Given the pathophysiology of SSc in other organ systems, it is not surprising that microvascular lesions and vasospasm are the likely causes of myocardial fibrosis in SSc.[66] The prevalence of conventional coronary artery disease is not increased in SSc but coronary vasospasm is more frequently seen, demonstrated by a decreased coronary reserve in patients with normal coronary arteries.[66] Reversible cold-induced perfusion defects have been described as "Raynaud's phenomenon of the heart."[70] This vasoreactivity may explain the beneficial cardiac effects of calcium-channel blockers in SSc. Because of superior resolution for subendocardial defects, cardiac MRI offers advantages over stress echocardiography or nuclear medicine scintigraphy for the evaluation of cardiac perfusion.[66]

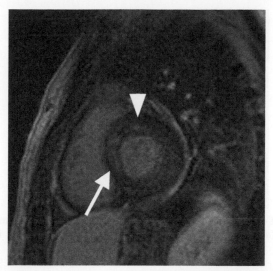

Fig. 25. Delayed postcontrast short-axis cardiac MR image at the level of the mid-portion of the heart shows patchy enhancement in the mid-septum (*arrow*) and anterior wall (*arrowhead*), consistent with fibrosis in SSc.

Diastolic Dysfunction

Cardiac diastolic dysfunction in SSc may be caused by myocardial fibrosis or pericardial disease, and is reported in up to 50% of patients with SSc.[71] Diastolic dysfunction is defined by impaired ventricular filling and compliance, with large pressure changes corresponding to a blunted ventricular volume response.[72] When heart failure manifests clinically with a normal ejection fraction, diastolic dysfunction is appropriately termed diastolic heart failure. Decreased flow velocities during early ventricular filling, elevated end-diastolic pressures, and prolonged relaxation are measures of reduced diastolic compliance.[73]

As for PH, DE is useful in evaluating for diastolic dysfunction in SSc.[74] On DE, measuring flow velocity across the mitral valve allows for the comparison of early (E) and late (A) diastolic filling velocities, as well as calculation of the isovolumetric relaxation time (IVRT) and the rate of deceleration in flow (DT). Early diastolic dysfunction is characterized by a decreased E/A ratio, and progressive diastolic dysfunction is characterized by a decrease in DT and IVRT.[73] On MRI, cardiac motion and blood flow are precisely evaluated by wall tagging and phase-contrast techniques.[73] Rubinshtein and colleagues[75] showed moderately good correlation between cardiac MRI and echocardiography for assessment of diastolic dysfunction parameters, and correctly identified 23 of 25 patients with restrictive dysfunction at echocardiography. Rathi and colleagues[76] also found good agreement between MRI and DE for evaluation of diastolic function.

Pericardial Disease

Pericardial manifestations of SSc include pericardial effusions and fibrous pericarditis. Whereas 30% to 70% of autopsy specimens show pericardial disease, only 5% to 15% of patients have symptoms.[67] Pericardial effusions may be a presentation of heart failure or PH in SSc.[67] Pericardial effusions are suggested by radiographic enlargement of the cardiac shadow and are readily confirmed by ultrasonography, CT, or MRI (**Fig. 26**). Postcontrast CT or MRI reveal enhancement surrounding a thickened pericardium or enhancing pericardial fluid in cases of pericarditis (**Fig. 27**).[77]

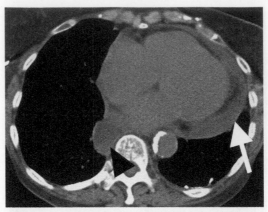

Fig. 26. CT without contrast demonstrates a pericardial effusion filling and distending the pericardial space (*arrow*). In addition, the esophagus is filled with fluid and dilated (*arrowhead*).

DE is a significant part of the algorithm for initial evaluation and follow-up of patients with SSc. Clinicians should be familiar with the capabilities of CT and DE for evaluation of primary cardiac involvement, PH, and pericardial disease in SSc patients (**Box 5**). With the capability to accurately evaluate cardiac function and flow as well as perfusion and fibrosis in a single session, cardiac MRI is likely to undergo increased use in SSc patients in the future.

GASTROINTESTINAL INVOLVEMENT IN SYSTEMIC SCLEROSIS

The GI tract is the second most common site of involvement in patients with SSc; only skin involvement is more frequent.[78] Symptomatic GI disease is present in 50% of patients.[79] Up to 10% of deaths in SSc may be attributed to GI disease.[78] Although GI involvement is more frequent in dcSSc patients, esophageal disease is also common in lcSSc.[79] As in other organ systems, the pathogenesis of disease in the GI tract is due to small-vessel endothelial proliferation, autonomic neural disturbance, and

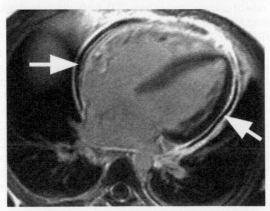

Fig. 27. Delayed postcontrast axial cardiac MR image shows thick high-signal enhancement deep and superficial to thickened low-signal pericardium (*arrows*). This appearance is consistent with pericarditis.

Box 5
Cardiac involvement in systemic sclerosis
Right heart overload caused by pulmonary hypertension
Myocardial fibrosis
Diastolic dysfunction
Pericardial effusion and pericarditis

fibrosis.[79] All portions of the GI tract from the esophagus to the anus may be involved. Although barium esophagography and enterography are the traditional methods for imaging the GI tract in SSc, ingested barium may exacerbate pseudo-obstruction caused by involvement of the small bowel. Therefore, CT or MR imaging of the bowel may be preferable.[10]

Upper GI Disease

Up to 90% of SSc patients have demonstrable esophageal motility abnormalities.[78] Barium esophagography allows for dynamic evaluation of esophageal motility. Absent peristaltic waves are noted in the lower two-thirds of the esophagus, but may also affect the striated muscle of the upper esophagus in advanced disease. The tone of the lower esophageal sphincter is decreased, resulting in a patulous appearance. As disease progresses, the esophagus appears dilated (**Fig. 28**). These findings are

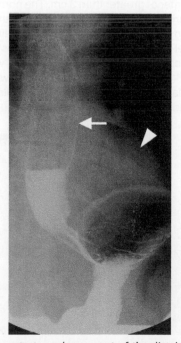

Fig. 28. Esophagogram demonstrates enlargement of the distal esophagus (*arrow*). Dynamically, there is decreased esophageal contraction consistent with dysmotility secondary to SSc. Increased interstitial markings secondary to pulmonary fibrosis are subtly noted in the left lower lobe (*arrowhead*).

most apparent when an esophagogram is performed in the recumbent, rather than standing, position.[80] When performed in a cohort with a 90% prevalence of abnormal manometric findings, barium esophagography demonstrated abnormal motility in 60% to 70% of cases.[81] On CT, esophageal dysmotility is diagnosed when the air-filled esophagus is greater than 10 mm in coronal diameter, contains a fluid level, or is filled with fluid.[82]

Gastroesophageal reflux may also be observed during barium esophagography. In turn, reflux leads to esophagitis, ulceration, and stricture formation.[80] The incidence of Barrett esophagus is increased in SSc, but the association with adenocarcinoma is less clear than in non-SSc patients.[78] Endoscopy allows for dilation of strictures and is indicated for surveillance in Barrett esophagus.

The stomach is the least common site of GI involvement with SSc, but delayed gastric emptying and gastric antral vascular ectasia (GAVE) may be present.[10] Although gastric dilation can be seen on radiographs or CT in advanced cases, delayed gastric emptying is best diagnosed by nuclear medicine scintigraphy that demonstrates abnormal retention of radiolabeled solids.[78] The telangiectasias of GAVE have the appearance of a "watermelon stomach" at endoscopy, and may lead to massive hemorrhage if untreated. Laser or argon coagulation treatments are effective but may have to be repeated.[78]

Bowel Disease

Fibrosis of the small bowel in SSc causes luminal dilation and longitudinal approxima-tion of the folds of the valvulae conniventes, creating a "hidebound" appearance.[83] Small-bowel dilation in SSc typically involves the duodenum or jejunum, and is char-acterized as a jejunal diameter of greater than 3 cm. The normal jejunum demonstrates 4 to 7 folds per inch on barium enterography or CT; more than 7 folds per inch or the preservation of normal fold spacing in the face of bowel dilation is consistent with a fibrosed, hidebound bowel (**Fig. 29**).[83] Asymmetric fibrosis of one side of the bowel wall results in pseudosacculation of the uninvolved side, which is characteristically the antimesenteric wall.[83] Involvement of the small bowel in SSc results in im-paired motility and bacterial overgrowth.[78] Small-bowel dilation and delayed motility cause the clinical and radiographic presentation of pseudo-obstruction. Bacterial

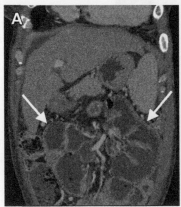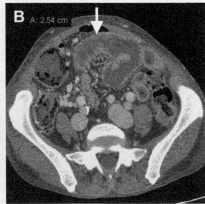

Fig. 29. CT of the abdomen with contrast in the coronal (*A*) and axial (*B*) planes demon-strates dilated loops of jejunum (*arrows*) measuring up to 5 cm in diameter. On the axial image (*B*), the jejunal mucosal folds appear crowded, and there are more than 7 folds over the indicated distance of 1 inch; this is the hidebound appearance of small bowel.

overgrowth and decreased motility can result in fecalization of the small bowel, which has been termed the "small bowel feces sign" (**Fig. 30**).[84]

Involvement of the colon in SSc is also characterized by fibrosis and dilation. Colonic pseudosacculations and pneumatosis intestinalis may be seen on CT.[10] Ano-rectal disease in SSc is in fact more common than involvement of the small or large bowel, and presents with incontinence. On MRI, ventral deviation of the anterior rectal wall, sphincter atrophy, and contrast enhancement of the sphincter consistent with fibrosis are seen (**Box 6**).[85]

RENAL INVOLVEMENT IN SYSTEMIC SCLEROSIS

Before the introduction of angiotensin-converting enzyme (ACE) inhibitors, sclero-derma renal crisis (SRC), normally presenting with acute hypertension, was the most deadly complication of SSc, with a 10% 1-year survival.[86] With ACE-inhibitor–based treatment, up to 60% of patients require no or only temporary dialysis.[86] SRC is reported in 10% of SSc patients and is approximately 10 times more common in dcSSC.[86,87] Other risk factors for SRC include high-dose (>15 mg/d) steroid use, the presence of a pericardial effusion, and the RNA polymerase III antibody.[86,87]

Similar to other organ systems, acute and insidious renal injury in scleroderma is mediated by small-vessel endothelial dysfunction and intimal proliferation and may be episodic in nature, similar to RP.[86] Chronic renal pathology is present in up to 80% of autopsy studies, and hypertension, proteinuria, and azotemia occur in 50% of SSc patients. However, these findings are relatively mild and often secondary to nonrenal causes.[86] One notable association is that between renal impairment and PAH.[87] In routine clinical evaluation of SSc, renal imaging plays a limited role. Radio-isotope renal scintigraphy with diethylenetriamine pentaacetic acid is useful for

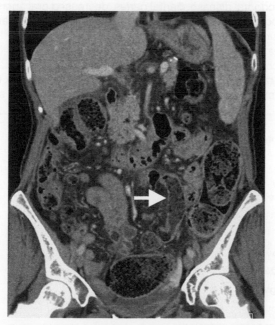

Fig. 30. Coronal contrast-enhanced abdomen CT shows fecal material in the mid-proximal small bowel (*arrow*) in a patient with SSc. The small-bowel feces sign can be seen secondary to delayed transit and/or bacterial overgrowth in patients with systemic sclerosis.

Box 6
Gastrointestinal involvement in systemic sclerosis

Lower esophageal dysmotility and dilation

Esophageal reflux and strictures

GAVE and delayed gastric emptying

Proximal small bowel dilated, hidebound, and sacculated

Fecalization of small bowel and colon

Anorectal fibrosis and thinning

---

measurement of glomerular filtration rate, and Doppler ultrasonography has been used to demonstrate decreases in the renal vascular resistance index (RI). Unlike in lupus, however, changes in renal RI in patients with SSc are not correlated with poor outcomes.[87] As with imaging in other organ systems, renal imaging may be useful as a surrogate marker in future trials in patients with SSc.

ORAL INVOLVEMENT IN SYSTEMIC SCLEROSIS

SSc commonly involves the facial and oral areas, leading to significant morbidity in this patient population. It is important to recognize the potential oral manifestations of SSc (**Box 7**). Given the importance of the mouth both functionally and aesthetically, poor oral health may significantly affect the lives of SSc patients.

Tongue rigidity and hardening of the facial skin and intraoral tissues are the most common oral manifestations of SSc, and lead to the characteristic facial features. Fibrosis of the orofacial complex may result in a variety of oral complications including microstomia, periodontal disease, dental caries, decreased oral aperture, mucogingival defects, temporomandibular disorder, trigeminal neuropathy, and other unique radiographic features.

Oral Imaging

There are several radiographic changes to the maxillofacial complex that can be seen in SSc. A uniform widening of the periodontal ligament (PDL) space has been

---

Box 7
Oral involvement in patients with systemic sclerosis

Xerostomia

Microstomia

Dental caries, periodontal disease

Enamel erosion

Dysphagia

Fibrosis of oral tissues

Mucosal telangiectasias

Trigeminal neuralgia

Mandibular resorption

Periodontal ligament space widening

Osteonecrosis of the jaw (possibly related to medication use)

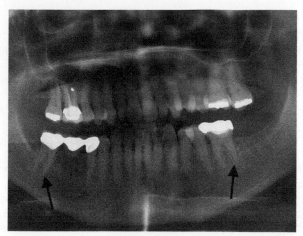

Fig. 31. Panorex dental image demonstrates uniform widening of the periodontal ligament space surrounding the mandibular molars (*arrows*).

described in up to 10% of patients with SSc.[88] This widening is related to fibrotic thickening of the PDL and is of no known clinical significance (**Fig. 31**).

Resorption of the coronoid process, condylar head, and angle of the mandible has been detected radiographically in 20% of SSc patients.[89] The resorption of bone is possibly related to increased pressure associated with abnormal collagen deposition in the adjacent oral facial tissues. Another potential cause of bone resorption is vascular ischemia, with the obstruction of small muscular vessels leading to muscle atrophy, which may contribute to the pressure of tight skin to the bone thereby affecting the blood supply to the bone itself. Severe resorption in the area of the mandibular angle may result in the "tail of the whale" pattern on dental radiographs. If severe enough, mandibular resorption increases the risk for pathologic fracture of the mandible in such patients with SSc.

Other imaging modalities have been used to assess the oral health in patients with SSc. A recent study used MRI to analyze the masseter musculature in patients with SSc.[90] The study investigated the relationship between mandibular osteolysis, MRI signal changes, and strength of the masseter muscle in 15 SSc patients. It was found that patients with SSc had increased fat replacement, rectification, and atrophy of the masseter muscle in comparison with controls. In addition, T2 signal on MRI was significantly increased among patients with SSc without osteolysis, compared with SSc patients with osteolysis and normal controls.[90]

Ultrasonography has also been used to assess the appearance of the oral mucosa in patients with SSc. In one study 20-MHz ultrasonography was performed, and patients with SSc were noted to have increased echogenicity attributable to fibrotic deposition.[91] Ultrasonography may be a valuable noninvasive means by which to evaluate fibrosis of the oral mucosa in patients with SSc.

SUMMARY

SSc is a rare connective tissue disease affecting multiple organ systems, and is associated with significant morbidity and mortality. Imaging is an important adjunct when screening and following patients for systemic involvement. The astute clinician must recognize the importance of detecting patients with SSc and the role of imaging in caring for these complex patients.

REFERENCES

1. Mayes MD, Reveille JD. Epidemiology, demographics and genetics. In: Clements PJ, Furst DE, editors. Systemic sclerosis. Philadelphia: Lippincott Williams and Wilkins; 2004. p. 1–15.
2. Hinchcliff M, Varga J. Systemic sclerosis/scleroderma: a treatable multisystem disease. Am Fam Physician 2008;78:961–8.
3. Hachulla E, Launay D. Diagnosis and classification of systemic sclerosis. Clin Rev Allergy Immunol 2011;40:78–83.
4. Strollo D, Goldin J. Imaging lung disease in systemic sclerosis. Curr Rheumatol Rep 2010;12:156–61.
5. Highland KB, Garin MC, Brown KK. The spectrum of scleroderma lung disease. Semin Respir Crit Care Med 2007;284:418–29.
6. LeRoy C, Black C, Fleischmajer R, et al. Scleroderma (systemic sclerosis): classification, subsets and pathogenesis. J Rheumatol 1988;15:202–5.
7. Steen VD. Autoantibodies in systemic sclerosis. Semin Arthritis Rheum 2005;351: 35–42.
8. Resnick D. Scleroderma. In: Resnick D, editor. Diagnosis of bone and joint disorders, vol. 2, 4th edition. Philadelphia: WB Saunders; 2002. p. 1194–220.
9. Block JA, Sequeira W. Raynaud's phenomenon. Lancet 2001;357:2042–8.
10. Madani G, Katz RD, Haddock JA, et al. The role of radiology in the management of systemic sclerosis. Clin Radiol 2008;639:959–67.
11. Kaldas M, Khanna PP, Furst DE, et al. Sensitivity to change of the modified Rodnan skin score in diffuse systemic sclerosis–assessment of individual body sites in two large randomized controlled trials. Rheumatology (Oxford) 2009;48: 1143–6.
12. Hesselstrand R, Scheja A, Wildt M, et al. High-frequency ultrasound of skin involvement in systemic sclerosis reflects oedema, extension and severity in early disease. Rheumatology (Oxford) 2008;47:84–7.
13. Schanz S, Henes J, Ulmer A, et al. Magnetic resonance imaging findings in patients with systemic scleroderma and musculoskeletal symptoms. Eur Radiol 2013;23:212–21.
14. Galluccio F, Matucci-Cerinic M. Two faces of the same coin: Raynaud phenomenon and digital ulcers in systemic sclerosis. Autoimmun Rev 2011;10: 241–3.
15. Avouac J, Guerini H, Wipff J, et al. Radiological hand involvement in systemic sclerosis. Ann Rheum Dis 2006;65:1088–92.
16. Yune HY, Vix VA, Klatte EC. Early fingertip changes in scleroderma. JAMA 1971; 215:1113–6.
17. Bassett LW, Blocka KL, Furst DE, et al. Skeletal findings in progressive systemic sclerosis (scleroderma). AJR Am J Roentgenol 1981;136:1121–6.
18. Erre GL, Marongiu A, Fenu P, et al. The "sclerodermic hand": a radiological and clinical study. Joint Bone Spine 2008;75:426–31.
19. Boutry N, Hachulla E, Zanetti-Musielak C, et al. Imaging features of musculoskeletal involvement in systemic sclerosis. Eur Radiol 2007;17:1172–80.
20. Steen VD, Medsger TA Jr. The palpable tendon friction rub: an important physical examination finding in patients with systemic sclerosis. Arthritis Rheum 1997;40: 1146–51.
21. Stoenoiu MS, Houssiau FA, Lecouvet FE. Tendon friction rubs in systemic sclerosis: a possible explanation–an ultrasound and magnetic resonance imaging study. Rheumatology (Oxford) 2013;52:529–33.

22. Randone SB, Guiducci S, Cerinic MM. Musculoskeletal involvement in systemic sclerosis. Best Pract Res Clin Rheumatol 2008;22:339–50.

23. Tagliafico A, Panico N, Serafini G, et al. The thickness of the A1 pulleys reflects the disability of hand mobility in scleroderma. A pilot study using high-frequency ultrasound. Eur J Radiol 2011;77:254–7.

24. La Montagna G, Sodano A, Capurro V, et al. The arthropathy of systemic sclerosis: a 12 month prospective clinical and imaging study. Skeletal Radiol 2005;34:5–41.

25. Blocka KL, Bassett LW, Furst DE, et al. The arthropathy of advanced progressive systemic sclerosis. A radiographic survey. Arthritis Rheum 1981;24:874–84.

26. Baron M, Lee P, Keystone EC. The articular manifestations of progressive systemic sclerosis (scleroderma). Ann Rheum Dis 1982;41:47–52.

27. Jinnin M, Ihn H, Yamane K, et al. Clinical features of patients with systemic sclerosis accompanied by rheumatoid arthritis. Clin Exp Rheumatol 2003;21:91–4.

28. Avouac J, Clements PJ, Khanna D, et al. Articular involvement in systemic sclerosis. Rheumatology (Oxford) 2012;51:1347–56.

29. Cuomo G, Zappia M, Abignano G, et al. Ultrasonographic features of the hand and wrist in systemic sclerosis. Rheumatology (Oxford) 2009;48:1414–7.

30. Generini S, Steiner G, Miniati I, et al. Anti-hnRNP and other autoantibodies in systemic sclerosis with joint involvement. Rheumatology (Oxford) 2009;48:920–5.

31. Low AH, Lax M, Johnson SR, et al. Magnetic resonance imaging of the hand in systemic sclerosis. J Rheumatol 2009;36:961–4.

32. Le Pavec J, Launay D, Mathai SC, et al. Scleroderma lung disease. Clin Rev Allergy Immunol 2011;40:104–16.

33. Kim DS, Yoo B, Lee JS, et al. The major histopathologic pattern of pulmonary fibrosis in scleroderma is nonspecific interstitial pneumonia. Sarcoidosis Vasc Diffuse Lung Dis 2002;19:121–7.

34. Desai SR, Veeraraghavan S, Hansell DM, et al. CT features of lung disease in patients with systemic sclerosis: comparison with idiopathic pulmonary fibrosis and nonspecific interstitial pneumonia. Radiology 2004;232:560–7.

35. Lynch DA, Travis WD, Muller NL, et al. Idiopathic interstitial pneumonias: CT features. Radiology 2005;236:10–21.

36. Kligerman SJ, Groshong S, Brown KK, et al. Nonspecific interstitial pneumonia: radiologic, clinical, and pathologic considerations. Radiographics 2009;29: 73–87.

37. Arakawa H, Honma K. Honeycomb lung: history and current concepts. AJR Am J Roentgenol 2011;196:773–82.

38. Schurawitzki H, Stiglbauer R, Graninger W, et al. Interstitial lung disease in progressive systemic sclerosis: high-resolution CT versus radiography. Radiology 1990;176:755–9.

39. Launay D, Remy-Jardin M, Michon-Pasturel U, et al. High resolution computed tomography in fibrosing alveolitis associated with systemic sclerosis. J Rheumatol 2006;33:1789–801.

40. Tashkin DP, Elashoff R, Clements PJ, et al. Cyclophosphamide versus placebo in scleroderma lung disease. N Engl J Med 2006;354:2655–66.

41. Goh NS, Desai SR, Veeraraghavan S, et al. Interstitial lung disease in systemic sclerosis: a simple staging system. Am J Respir Crit Care Med 2008;177: 1248–54.

42. Bouros D, Wells AU, Nicholson AG, et al. Histopathologic subsets of fibrosing alveolitis in patients with systemic sclerosis and their relationship to outcome. Am J Respir Crit Care Med 2002;165:1581–6.

43. Strange C, Bolster MB, Roth MD, et al. Bronchoalveolar lavage and response to cyclophosphamide in scleroderma interstitial lung disease. Am J Respir Crit Care Med 2008;177:91–8.

44. Lee KS, Kullnig P, Hartman TE, et al. Cryptogenic organizing pneumonia: CT findings in 43 patients. AJR Am J Roentgenol 1994;162:543–6.

45. Rossi SE, Erasmus JJ, McAdams HP, et al. Pulmonary drug toxicity: radiologic and pathologic manifestations. Radiographics 2000;20:1245–59.

46. Thompson AE, Pope JE. A study of the frequency of pericardial and pleural effusions in scleroderma. Br J Rheumatol 1998;37:1320–3.

47. Franquet T, Gimenez A, Roson N, et al. Aspiration diseases: findings, pitfalls, and differential diagnosis. Radiographics 2000;20:673–85.

48. McLaughlin V, Humbert M, Coghlan G, et al. Pulmonary arterial hypertension: the most devastating vascular complication of systemic sclerosis. Rheumatology (Oxford) 2009;48(S3):iii25–31.

49. Chang B, Schachna L, White B, et al. Natural history of mild-moderate pulmonary hypertension and the risk factors for severe pulmonary hypertension in scleroderma. J Rheumatol 2006;33:269–74.

50. Denton CP, Cailes JB, Phillips GD, et al. Comparison of Doppler echocardiography and right heart catheterization to assess pulmonary hypertension in systemic sclerosis. Br J Rheumatol 1997;36:239–43.

51. Castaner E, Gallardo X, Ballesteros E, et al. CT diagnosis of chronic pulmonary thromboembolism. Radiographics 2009;29:31–50.

52. Ridge CA, Bankier AA, Eisenberg RL. Mosaic attenuation. AJR Am J Roentgenol 2011;197:W970–7.

53. Grosse C, Grosse A. CT findings in diseases associated with pulmonary hypertension: a current review. Radiographics 2010;30:1753–77.

54. Yeh BM, Kurzman P, Foster E, et al. Clinical relevance of retrograde inferior vena cava or hepatic vein opacification during contrast-enhanced CT. AJR Am J Roentgenol 2004;183:1227–32.

55. Tan RT, Kuzo R, Goodman LR, et al. Utility of CT scan evaluation for predicting pulmonary hypertension in patients with parenchymal lung disease. Medical College of Wisconsin Lung Transplant Group. Chest 1998;113:1250–6.

56. Ng CS, Wells AU, Padley SP. A CT sign of chronic pulmonary arterial hypertension: the ratio of main pulmonary artery to aortic diameter. J Thorac Imaging 1999;14:270–8.

57. Alhamad EH, Al-Boukai AA, Al-Kassimi FA, et al. Prediction of pulmonary hypertension in patients with or without interstitial lung disease: reliability of CT findings. Radiology 2011;260:875–83.

58. Wieben O, Francois C, Reeder SB. Cardiac MRI of ischemic heart disease at 3 T: potential and challenges. Eur J Radiol 2008;65:15–28.

59. Haddad F, Hunt SA, Rosenthal DN, et al. Right ventricular function in cardiovascular disease, part I: anatomy, physiology, aging, and functional assessment of the right ventricle. Circulation 2008;117:1436–48.

60. Benza R, Biederman R, Murali S, et al. Role of cardiac magnetic resonance imaging in the management of patients with pulmonary arterial hypertension. J Am Coll Cardiol 2008;52:1683–92.

61. Roeleveld RJ, Marcus JT, Faes TJ, et al. Interventricular septal configuration at MR imaging and pulmonary arterial pressure in pulmonary hypertension. Radiology 2005;234:710–7.

62. Blyth KG, Groenning BA, Martin TN, et al. Contrast enhanced-cardiovascular magnetic resonance imaging in patients with pulmonary hypertension. Eur Heart J 2005;26:1993–9.

63. McCann GP, Gan CT, Beek AM, et al. Extent of MRI delayed enhancement of myocardial mass is related to right ventricular dysfunction in pulmonary artery hypertension. AJR Am J Roentgenol 2007;188:349–55.

64. Junqueira FP, Macedo R, Coutinho AC, et al. Myocardial delayed enhancement in patients with pulmonary hypertension and right ventricular failure: evaluation by cardiac MRI. Br J Radiol 2009;82:821–6.

65. Tzelepis GE, Kelekis NL, Plastiras SC, et al. Pattern and distribution of myocardial fibrosis in systemic sclerosis: a delayed enhanced magnetic resonance imaging study. Arthritis Rheum 2007;56:3827–36.

66. Kahan A, Allanore Y. Primary myocardial involvement in systemic sclerosis. Rheumatology (Oxford) 2006;45(S4):iv14–7.

67. Champion HC. The heart in scleroderma. Rheum Dis Clin North Am 2008;34: 181–90.

68. Hassan WM, Fawzy ME, Al Helaly S, et al. Pitfalls in diagnosis and clinical, echocardiographic, and hemodynamic findings in endomyocardial fibrosis: a 25-year experience. Chest 2005;128:3985–92.

69. Carette S, Turcotte J, Mathon G. Severe myositis and myocarditis in progressive systemic sclerosis. J Rheumatol 1985;12:997–9.

70. Lekakis J, Mavrikakis M, Emmanuel M, et al. Cold-induced coronary Raynaud's phenomenon in patients with systemic sclerosis. Clin Exp Rheumatol 1998;16: 135–40.

71. Nakajima K, Taki J, Kawano M, et al. Diastolic dysfunction in patients with systemic sclerosis detected by gated myocardial perfusion SPECT: an early sign of cardiac involvement. J Nucl Med 2001;42:183–8.

72. Zile MR, Brutsaert DL. New concepts in diastolic dysfunction and diastolic heart failure: part I: diagnosis, prognosis, and measurements of diastolic function. Circulation 2002;105:1387–93.

73. van Kraaij DJ, van Pol PE, Ruiters AW, et al. Diagnosing diastolic heart failure. Eur J Heart Fail 2002;4:419–30.

74. Lanier GM, Vaishnava P, Kosmas CE, et al. An update on diastolic dysfunction. Cardiol Rev 2012;20:230–6.

75. Rubinshtein R, Glockner JF, Feng D, et al. Comparison of magnetic resonance imaging versus Doppler echocardiography for the evaluation of left ventricular diastolic function in patients with cardiac amyloidosis. Am J Cardiol 2009;103:718–23.

76. Rathi VK, Doyle M, Yamrozik J, et al. Routine evaluation of left ventricular diastolic function by cardiovascular magnetic resonance: a practical approach. J Cardiovasc Magn Reson 2008;10:36.

77. Wang ZJ, Reddy GP, Gotway MB, et al. CT and MR imaging of pericardial disease. Radiographics 2003;23(Spec No):S167–80.

78. Forbes A, Marie I. Gastrointestinal complications: the most frequent internal complications of systemic sclerosis. Rheumatology (Oxford) 2009;48(S3):iii36–9.

79. Sjogren RW. Gastrointestinal motility disorders in scleroderma. Arthritis Rheum 1994;37:1265–82.

80. Meszaros WT. The regional manifestations of scleroderma. Radiology 1958;70: 313–25.

81. Weihrauch TR, Korting GW. Manometric assessment of oesophageal involvement in progressive systemic sclerosis, morphoea and Raynaud's disease. Br J Dermatol 1982;107:325–32.

82. Bhalla M, Silver RM, Shepard JA, et al. Chest CT in patients with scleroderma: prevalence of asymptomatic esophageal dilatation and mediastinal lymphadenopathy. AJR Am J Roentgenol 1993;161:269–72.

83. Levine MS, Rubesin SE, Laufer I. Pattern approach for diseases of mesenteric small bowel on barium studies. Radiology 2008;249:445–60.
84. Fuchsjager MH. The small-bowel feces sign. Radiology 2002;225:378–9.
85. deSouza NM, Williams AD, Wilson HJ, et al. Fecal incontinence in scleroderma: assessment of the anal sphincter with thin-section endoanal MR imaging. Radiology 1998;208:529–35.
86. Steen VD. Scleroderma renal crisis. Rheum Dis Clin North Am 2003;29:315–33.
87. Shanmugam VK, Steen VD. Renal manifestations in scleroderma: evidence for subclinical renal disease as a marker of vasculopathy. Int J Rheumatol 2010; 2010. pii: 538589.
88. Greenburg M, Glick M. Immunologic diseases. In: Ciarroca K, Greenburg M, editors. Burket's oral medicine. Hamilton (Ontario): BC Decker; 2003. p. 491–4.
89. Neville B, Damm D, Allen C, et al. Dermatologic diseases. In: Neville B, Damm D, Allen C, et al, editors. Oral and maxillofacial pathology. Philadelphia: WB Saunders; 1995. p. 585–7.
90. Marcucci M, Abdala N. Analysis of the masseter muscle in patients with systemic sclerosis: a study by magnetic resonance imaging. Dentomaxillofac Radiol 2009; 38:524–30.
91. Jackowski J, Jöhren P, Müller AM, et al. Imaging of fibrosis of the oral mucosa by 20 MHz sonography. Dentomaxillofac Radiol 1999;28:290–4.

Imaging of Rheumatoid Arthritis

Lisa C. Vasanth, MD, MSc[a],*, Helene Pavlov, MD[b],
Vivian Bykerk, BSc, MD, FRCPC[c]

KEYWORDS

- Rheumatoid arthritis • Imaging • Radiography

KEY POINTS

- Increased awareness of the need for early diagnosis of rheumatoid arthritis and advances in the ability to effectively treat rheumatoid arthritis have made disease remission and maintenance of function a reality for many patients.
- Imaging plays a significant role in the diagnosis of rheumatoid arthritis, the determination of remission, and follow-up to monitor for progressive joint damage.
- Conventional radiographs of hands and feet remain the most commonly used method to assess joint damage and monitor disease progression in rheumatoid arthritis.
- Ultrasound allows assessment of synovitis, tenosynovitis, enthesitis, and erosions.
- Magnetic resonance imaging has the potential to directly visualize articular hyaline cartilage and to evaluate volume, thickness, morphology, and structural integrity.

Early identification and early treatment with disease modifying antirheumatic drugs (DMARDs) has become the standard of care for patients with rheumatoid arthritis. The goals are to alleviate symptoms, maintain and improve function, and prevent structural damage. Progression of structural damage has been associated with loss of function.[1] Imaging plays a significant role in the diagnosis of rheumatoid arthritis, the determination of remission, and follow-up to monitor for progressive joint damage.

RADIOGRAPHS

Despite the advent of ultrasound and magnetic resonance imaging (MRI), conventional radiographs of hands and feet remain the most commonly used method to

Funding Sources: None.
Conflict of Interest: L.C. Vasanth, has none. H. Pavlov developed an online course for Phillips Medical System. V. Bykerk has consulted for Antares, Astellas, Amgen, Pfizer, BMS, UCB, Roche, and Genentech.
[a] Department of Rheumatology, Weill Cornell Medical College, Hospital for Special Surgery, 525 East 71st Street, 7th Floor, New York, NY 10021, USA; [b] Department of Radiology, Weill Cornell Medical College, Hospital for Special Surgery, 535 East 70th Street, New York, NY 10021, USA; [c] Department of Rheumatology, Hospital for Special Surgery, 525 East 71st Street, 7th Floor, New York, NY 10021, USA
* Corresponding author.
E-mail address: vasanthl@hss.edu

Rheum Dis Clin N Am 39 (2013) 547–566
http://dx.doi.org/10.1016/j.rdc.2013.03.007
0889-857X/13/$ – see front matter © 2013 Elsevier Inc. All rights reserved.

rheumatic.theclinics.com

assess joint damage and monitor disease progression in rheumatoid arthritis. Radiographs are readily available, cost-effective, and have good reproducibility.[2] Radiographic signs of rheumatoid arthritis include soft tissue swelling, joint effusions, juxta-articular osteopenia, uniform joint space narrowing, cysts, bone erosions, joint subluxations, and malalignment.[3] Changes in the second to fifth metatarsophalangeal joints of the feet often appear before changes are noted in the hands.[4] The metacarpophalangeal (MCP) and proximal interphalangeal joints are most commonly affected in the hands, whereas the ulnar styloid joint is the most common site for erosions in the wrist.[4]

Scoring systems have developed to standardize the assessment of radiographic damage in evaluating rheumatoid arthritis. Most systems focus on the hands and feet because damage in the hands and feet is highly correlated with overall joint damage.[5] The most widely used scoring systems are the Sharp/van der Heijde (SvdH) method, the Larsen method, and the Sharp/Genant method.[6,7] The SvdH method assesses erosions and joint space narrowing separately, and it can be used for both hand and foot films.[8] The Genant/Sharp method focuses on 14 sites for erosions and 13 sites for joint space narrowing for a maximum score of 100.[9] The Larsen system uses reference films to assess the joint and grades joint involvement largely based on erosions.[8]

SVDH SCORING METHOD

With the SvdH method, erosions are assessed in 16 joints for each hand and wrist, and 6 joints for each foot.[10] Erosions are graded as follows: 0, no erosions; 1, discrete; 2, larger; 3, extending to the imaginary middle of the bone; 4+, erosions extending over the imaginary middle of the bone; and 5, extensive.[10] Joint space narrowing is assessed in 15 areas for each hand and wrist and 6 areas for each foot.[10] Joint space narrowing is scored as follows: 0, normal; 1, focal; 2, generalized (>50% of the original joint space left); 3, generalized (<50% of the original joint space is left or there this subluxation); 4, bony ankylosis or complete subluxation.[10] The erosion score ranges from 0 to 160 for the hands and wrists and 0 to 120 for the feet. The joint space narrowing score ranges from 0 to 120 for the hands and wrists and 0 to 48 for the feet. Therefore, the total SvdH score ranges from 0 to 448 (**Fig. 1**).[10]

THE SIMPLIFIED EROSION NARROWING SCORE

The Sharp method and the SvdH method both require trained and experienced readers to ensure reliable scores. As a result, Dias and colleagues[11] proposed a simplified method, the Simplified Erosion Narrowing Score (SENS), which could feasibly be used to assess structural damage in clinical practice and compared it with the SvdH method. The SENS method assesses erosions and joint space narrowing (JSN) in the same joints as the SvdH method, but instead of grading severity it only scores the presence or absence of erosions or JSN.[12] The study concluded that results of the SENS method correlated with those of the SvdH method and that the SENS method could potentially be validated for use in clinical practice.[12]

ROLE OF IMAGING AS AN OUTCOME MEASURE IN CLINICAL TRIALS

Radiographs show cumulative damage and, therefore, can be used to evaluate the effectiveness of treatment.[8] The Sharp score and SvdH score have been used as outcome measures in multiple large clinical trials, as outlined in **Table 1**.

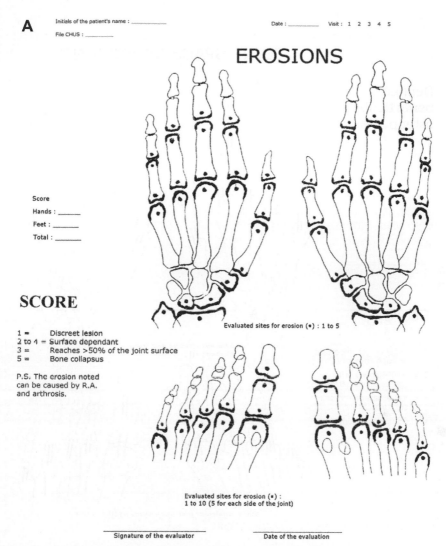

Initials of the patient's name : _____

File CHUS : _____

Date : _____ Visit : 1 2 3 4 5

EROSIONS

Score

Hands : _____

Feet : _____

Total : _____

SCORE

1 =   Discreet lesion
2 to 4 = Surface dependant
3 =   Reaches >50% of the joint surface
5 =   Bone collapsus

P.S. The erosion noted
can be caused by R.A.
and arthrosis.

Evaluated sites for erosion (•) : 1 to 5

Evaluated sites for erosion (•) :
1 to 10 (5 for each side of the joint)

Signature of the evaluator   Date of the evaluation

Fig. 1. (*A, B*) With the SvdH method, erosions are assessed in 16 joints for each hand and wrist, and 6 joints for each foot. RA, Rheumatoid arthritis. (*Adapted from* Hulsmans HM, Jacobs JW, van der Heijde DM, et al. The course of radiologic damage during the first six years of rheumatoid arthritis. Arthritis Rheum 2000;43(9):1929; with permission.)

INTERPRETING RADIOGRAPHIC PROGRESSION

As noted in **Table 1**, clinical trials use different primary end points to assess treatment efficacy. In 2002, Bruynesteyn and colleagues[22] worked to define the relationship between the smallest detectable difference (SDD) noted on radiographs using the SvdH score and the minimal clinically important difference (MCID). The SDD is the smallest change in a scoring method that can reliably be differentiated from measurement error[22]; however, a statistical difference may not be clinically relevant. Five expert rheumatologists reviewed 46 pairs of hand and foot films for progression of joint

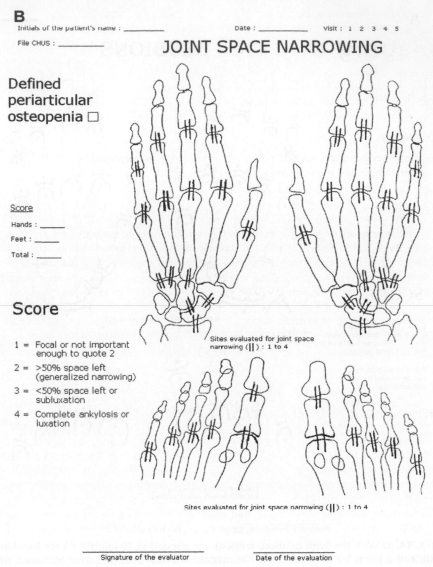

B

JOINT SPACE NARROWING

Defined periarticular osteopenia ☐

Score

Hands : _____

Feet : _____

Total : _____

Score

1 = Focal or not important enough to quote 2

2 = >50% space left (generalized narrowing)

3 = <50% space left or subluxation

4 = Complete ankylosis or luxation

Sites evaluated for joint space narrowing (‖) : 1 to 4

Sites evaluated for joint space narrowing (‖) : 1 to 4

_____   _____
Signature of the evaluator   Date of the evaluation

Fig. 1. (continued)

damage[22] and determined whether the progression in joint damage warranted change in treatment. The SDD for the SvdH score was 5, which correlated in this study with the radiographic change that causes an expert rheumatologist to change treatment (ie, the MCID).[22] Another way to report the data is to calculate the percentage of patients with progression of joint damage beyond a cutoff.[23] An international consensus group suggested a percentage of patients with progression greater than 0.5 for 2 observers or greater than 0 for 1 observer; or percentage of patients with progression greater than SDD.[24] Other groups have proposed the use of probability plots as outcome measures because only a small percentage of patients show radiographic progression and, therefore, the results are not normally distributed.[25] Probability plots show data in a continuous manner so readers can visualize the coherence of the data.[23] The SDD can be added to the plot, or readers can apply other cutoff points.[23]

Landewe and van der Heijde[25] used data from the Combinatietherapie Bij Reuma-toide Artritis (COBRA) trial to show the usefulness of probability plots. The COBRA was a randomized, double-blind, placebo-controlled trial of 155 patients with rheuma-toid arthritis for less than 2 years.[13] The trial compared treatment with sulfasalazine monotherapy and treatment with combination therapy (prednisone, methotrexate, and sulfasalazine).[13] Their graphs, shown in **Fig. 2**, show the progression scores for all the patients in the trial. It is easy to visualize the number of patients with no change in SvdH score as well as the number of patients with high scores who may shift the mean and standard deviation for the group.[25] It is easy to visualize the median, 25th, and 75th percentiles (see **Fig. 2**).[25]

Landewe and van der Heijde[25] also used probability plots to visually compare the results in the two treatment arms of the COBRA trial (**Fig. 3**). In **Fig. 3**, the radiographic progression of the treatment groups are compared (monotherapy shown in circles and combination therapy shown with triangles). The plots also show the importance of choice of cutoff level.[25] If the cutoff level is 0 and everyone with a score greater than 0 is considered to have progressed, the treatments would not be considered different (contrast of 7%).[25] If a progression of 5 Sharp units is considered the cutoff, the treatment contrast is 27%.[25]

WHEN DOES RADIOGRAPHIC DAMAGE CAUSE A CHANGE IN FUNCTION?

The Health Assessment Questionnaire (HAQ) is a patient measure of functional status that is used to assess disability in rheumatoid arthritis. A review by Scott and col-leagues[26] found that, in patients with early rheumatoid arthritis, average HAQ scores are about 25% of the maximum, a score largely driven by pain and synovitis, not joint damage. The effect of pain and synovitis on functional status seems to decline as damage increases. Scott and colleagues[26] noted a linear relationship of disability and damage when radiologic scores exceed 33% of maximal damage. Smolen and colleagues[27] used clinical trial data to estimate the level of disability related to 1 Sharp score unit. Because radiographic progression is not always linear, this estimation ap-plies on the group level. They estimated that the HAQ increases by one-tenth of a unit for every 10-unit increase in Sharp score.[27] In a systematic review of the literature, Bombardier and colleagues[1] found that evidence joint damage measured by Sharp or Larsen score correlated with physical disability as measured by HAQ, Arthritis Impact Measurement Scale, grip strength, Short Form 36 (SF-36), work disability, and quality of life. An increase in joint damage was associated with an increase in future disability over time.[1]

ARE CLINICAL MEASURES OF LOW DISEASE ACTIVITY OR REMISSION CORRELATED WITH RADIOGRAPHIC PROGRESSION?

The Swedish Pharmacotherapy (SWEFOT) trial studied the 2-year clinical and radio-logical outcomes of patients with early rheumatoid arthritis who achieved low Disease Activity Score 28 (DAS28; $\leq$3.2) with methotrexate monotherapy.[28] Most of the pa-tients remained on methotrexate (target dose 20 mg/wk) for the duration of the 2-year trial. At baseline, 48.1% of the 147 patients had no radiographic damage (SvdH score of 0), at 1 year this proportion had decreased to 26.9%, and at 2 years to 20.2%.[28] The mean progression after 2 years in patients who had follow-up radio-graphs (n = 101) was 3.9 (standard deviation = 6.84) (P = .0003).[28] There was no

Table 1
The role of imaging as an outcome measure in clinical trials

	Year	Subjects	Design	Treatment Groups	Outcome Measures	Sharp or SvdH Score
COBRA[13]	1997	N = 155 RA<2 y	Randomized double-blind, placebo-controlled 28-wk trial with step-down therapy through week 56 and observation through week 80	1. SSA 2. SSA + prednisone + methotrexate Taper: prednisone tapered first, then methotrexate	Primary outcome 1. Pool index of measures[a] 2. Change in SvdH score	Median change (range) at 28 wk: Combined group Erosions 0 (0–24) Narrowing 0 (0–11) Total 1 (0–28) SSZ group Erosions 4 (0–26) Narrowing 1 (0–20) Total 4 (0–28) Statistically significant change that persisted to week 80
Enbrel ERA Trial[14]	2002	N = 632 RA ≤ 3 y MTX naive +RF ≥ 3 erosions on radiograph	Randomized double-blind, placebo-controlled 1-y trial with 1-y open-label extension	1. Enbrel 10 mg BIW 2. Enbrel 25 mg BIW 3. MTX 7.5 mg Qwk increased to 20 mg Qwk as needed	Primary outcome 1. ACR 20, ACR50, ACR70 2. Change in Sharp score	Sharp score 1. At 2 y, mean change in total score from baseline: 25 mg Enbrel 1.3 units vs 3.2 units in the MTX group (P = .001) 2. Mean change in erosion score: 0.7 and 1.9 in 25 mg Enbrel and MTX group respectively (P = .017) 3. 63% of 25 mg Enbrel patients had no increase in total Sharp score vs 51% patients on MTX (P = .017) 4. 70% of 25 mg patients on Enbrel vs 58% of patients on MTX had no increase in erosions (P = .012)

				Primary outcome	SvdH score
TICORA[15]	2004	N = 111 RA<5 y DAS28>2.4	1. Intensive management 2. Usual care Both groups used sequential DMARDs	1. Mean decrease in DAS 2. Percentage of patients with good response Secondary outcome SvdH score	1. Mean change in total score in intensive group 4.5 (1–9.875) and routine group 4.5 (1.5–9) P = .02 2. Mean change in erosion score. Intensive group 0.5 (0–3.375) and routine group 3 (0.5–8.5) P = .002 3. Mean change in JSN in intensive group 3.25 (1.125–7.5) and routine group 8.5 (2–15.5) P = .331
ASPIRE[16]	2004	N = 1049 1. RA ≥ 3 mo and ≤3 y 2. ≥10 swollen and ≥12 tender joints 3. +RF, erosions, or CRP≥2.0 4. MTX and anti-TNF naive	3 groups in a 4:5:5 ratio 1. MTX-placebo 2. MTX + 3 ɯg/kg infliximab 3. MTX + 6 ɯg/kg infliximab	Primary outcomes 1. ACR N 2. Change in SvdH score at 54 wk 3. Change from baseline in HAQ scores averaged over weeks 30–54	SvdH score 1. Mean change in total score from baseline to week 54 in MTX vs 3 mg/kg infliximab vs 6 mg/kg infliximab 3.7 ± 9.6, 0.4 ± 5.8, 0.5 ± 5.6; P = .001 2. Mean change in erosion score 3.0 ± 7.8, 0.6 ± 4.9, 0.1 ± 4.2; P<.001

(continued on next page)

Table 1
(continued)

	Year	Subjects	Design	Treatment Groups	Outcome Measures	Sharp or SvdH Score
BeSt Study[17]	2005	N = 508 1. RA<2 y 2. Active disease	2-y multicenter, randomized, single-blind trial	1. Sequential DMARD monotherapy 2. Step-up combination therapy 3. Initial combination DMARD therapy with tapered high-dose prednisone 4. Initial combination DMARD therapy with infliximab	Primary outcomes 1. Functional ability by D-HAQ[18] 2. Change in SvdH score Secondary outcomes 1. ACR20, ACR50, and ACR70 2. Clinical remission DAS44<1.6	SvdH score Patients treated with initial combination therapy including prednisone (group 3) or infliximab (group 4) had significantly less progression of radiographic joint damage than did patients with sequential monotherapy (group 1) or step-up combination therapy (group 2). Median increases in total SvdH score were 2.0, 2.5, 1.0, and 0.5 in groups 1–4 respectively Number of patients without progression of total SvdH score (greater than the SDD) was higher in groups 3 and 4 than in groups 1 and 2: 76/114, 82/112, 104/120, 113/121 in groups 1–4 respectively

Trial	Year	Inclusion	Study Design	Treatment Arms	End Points	Results
PREMIER[19]	2006	N = 799 1. RA<3 y 2. Active disease	2-y multicenter, double-blind, active comparator–controlled phase III trial	1. Adalimumab + MTX 2. Adalimumab 3. Oral MTX	Primary end points 1. Percentage of patients with ACR50 at 1 y 2. Mean change from baseline in total SvdH score	SvdH score Mean change in total score at 1 y combination therapy 1.3 units vs adalimumab monotherapy 3.0 units (P = .002) vs MTX monotherapy 5.7 units (P<.001)
COMET[20]	2008	N = 542 1. MTX naïve 2. RA 3–24 mo 3. Active disease	24-mo double-blind, randomized, parallel-group, multicenter trial	1. MTX alone 2. MTX + etanercept	Primary end points 1. Remission by DAS28 2. Change in total SvdH score	SvdH score No change in SvdH score 125/230 (54%) in MTX and 184/246 (75%) in etanercept + MTX P<.001
RAPID 1[21]	2008	N = 982	52-wk randomized, double-blind, parallel-treatment trial	1. MTX alone 2. Certolizumab 400 mg Q2 wk 3. Certolizumab 200 mg Q2 wk	Primary end points 1. ACR20 at week 24 2. Mean change in baseline SvdH score at week 52	SvdH score Mean radiographic progression in 200-mg certolizumab group (0.4 Sharp units), 400-mg certolizumab (0.2 Sharp units), MTX alone (2.8 units) (P<.001 by rank analysis)

a Tender joint count, physician global, grip strength, ESR, McMaster Toronto Arthritis Questionnaire.

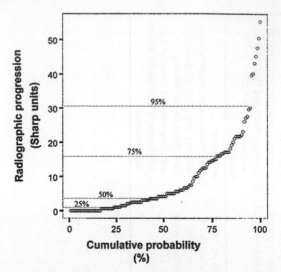

Fig. 2. Cumulative probability plot of the individual progression scores of 135 rheumatoid arthritis patients who participated in the COBRA trial. (*Data from* Landewe R, van der Heijde D. Radiographic progression depicted by probability plots: presenting data with optimal use of individual values. Arthritis Rheum 2004;50(3):701.)

statistically significant difference in progression between patients in DAS28 remission (DAS28<2.6) versus those not in remission (*P* = .73).[28]

Comparing radiographic outcomes with clinical outcomes can be problematic because patients in a clinical trial often show no radiographic progression during the trial and the few patients who show significant progression skew the results.[23]

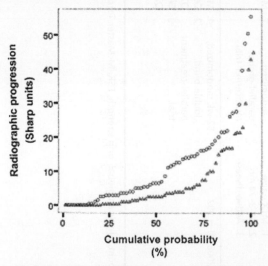

Fig. 3. Cumulative probability plots of individual 1-year radiographic progression scores in 135 rheumatoid arthritis patients who participated in the COBRA trial (67 patients in the monotherapy group [circles] and 68 patients in the combination therapy group [triangles]). Cumulative probability was calculated per group. (*Data from* Landewe R, van der Heijde D. Radiographic progression depicted by probability plots: presenting data with optimal use of individual values. Arthritis Rheum 2004;50(3):704.)

Missing data also make it difficult to compare clinical and radiographic outcomes.[29] Landewe and colleagues[29] showed that radiographic progression is often driven by a small number of patients who do not respond to treatment.

CAN RADIOGRAPHIC PROGRESSION HELP TO REDEFINE REMISSION?

Pain control, maintenance of physical function, and prevention of joint damage are important goals for treatment. The DAS28 is a clinical tool that uses tender and swollen joint counts, ESR, and patient global assessment to define disease activity and remission in patients with rheumatoid arthritis.[30] Investigators have questioned the DAS28 definition of remission because a significant number of patients in remission continue to have persistent joint swelling.[30] Aletaha and colleagues[31] analyzed data from the methotrexate monotherapy arms of the Active-Controlled Study of Patients Receiving Infliximab for the Treatment of Rheumatoid Arthritis of Early Onset (ASPIRE),[16] Trial of Adalimumab versus Methotrexate versus Combination of Adalimumab and Methotrexate in early rheumatoid arthritis (PREMIER),[19] Early Rheumatoid Arthritis trial of etanercept versus methotrexate,[32] Trial of Etanercept and Methotrexate with Radiographic Patient Outcomes (TEMPO),[33] and trials of leflunomide compared with sulfasalazine or methotrexate[34] and showed that patients on methotrexate monotherapy in DAS28 remission without joint swelling had lower rates of radiographic progression that those on methotrexate monotherapy who had persistent joint swelling.[31] Gandjbakhch and colleagues[35] evaluated 294 patients with rheumatoid arthritis who were in clinical remission or low disease activity state and found MRI evidence of subclinical inflammation (synovitis or bone edema) in many of the patients in clinical remission or with low disease activity states, which could explain radiographic progression in patients who are clinically doing well.[35]

Other studies by Landewe and colleagues[36] and Smolen and colleagues[37] have suggested a disconnect between clinically active disease and radiographic progression by documenting patients treated with methotrexate and anti–tumor necrosis factors who have persistent synovitis without radiographic progression. This phenomenon has also been seen with the COBRA strategy of step-down prednisolone[38] and with tocilizumab.[39] The disconnect may arise because clinical and radiographic findings are more likely caused by radiographic insensitivity and suggest that ultrasound and newer MRI techniques are more sensitive and better predictors of disease state. These results show the importance of evaluating both clinical and radiographic outcomes for patients who are treated with biologics.[40]

IS RADIOGRAPHIC EVIDENCE OF DISEASE PROGRESSION REVERSIBLE?

Remission is now the goal of treatment in rheumatoid arthritis. Lillegraven and colleagues[41] found that adding sustainability or time in clinical remission as a variable for rheumatoid arthritis remission criteria helped identify patients with a good future outcome (ie, no radiographic progression).

Is repair of joint damage possible? Improvement in SvdH scores has also been seen in clinical trials,[32,42] and case reports suggest that healing of erosions occasionally occurs.[43,44] However, changes can be subtle and healing of erosions can be difficult to differentiate from artifact or changes in positioning.[45]

ULTRASOUND AND MRI

Although radiographs are readily available and reproducible, they do not provide the earliest assessments of joint damage and cannot document bone edema or synovitis.[46] Early cartilage changes are not readily evident on radiographs because detection depends on indirect evidence shown as JSN. As a result, radiographs cannot reliably guide treatment decisions for patients with very early rheumatoid arthritis to the same degree as direct cartilage assessment, which is possible with cartilage-sensitive protocols on MRI or ultrasound. However, because of a lack of equipment and user standardization, uniform protocols for monitoring early rheumatoid arthritis or imaging changes after treatment are not yet established. Baillet and colleagues[47] reported that ultrasound was comparable with MRI and more effective than radiographs for diagnosing erosions. The Outcomes Measures in Rheumatoid Arthritis Clinical Trials (OMERACT) group defined ultrasound criteria for joint synovitis and erosions.[48] The European League Against Rheumatism (EULAR) and OMERACT are in the process of developing a global sonography scoring system specific for small-joint evaluation using gray-scale and power Doppler scores.[48,49]

Ultrasound

Ultrasound is a low-cost imaging modality that does not use ionizing radiation. Ultrasound allows assessment of synovitis, tenosynovitis, enthesitis, and erosions.[50] Transducers generate ultrasound pulses and receive returning echoes that are processed to form an anatomic image. The limitation of ultrasound in the musculoskeletal setting is that scans and technique are operator dependent[50] and it does not easily assess cartilage.[51] Portable devices are available but the degree of sensitivity for the detection of subtle changes varies with different ultrasound units and transducers. Normal hyaline cartilage is identified as anechoic (black, without echoes), hypoechoic (dark, few echoes), and a sharp interface with the subchondral bone.[51,52] When cartilage is not normal, the image is hyperechoic (bright with many echoes) along with a loss of the sharp interface with the subchondral bone.[51,52] High-end units with increased diagnostic accuracy and sensitivity will better enable detection of early rheumatoid disorders.[53] Power Doppler ultrasound records vascularity.[52] Active synovitis detected by power Doppler has been correlated with disease activity measured by DAS28 and radiographic progression.[54]

MRI

MRI uses a powerful magnetic field, applied in pulses, to detect water protons present in body tissue.[55] Limitations of MRI include cost, accessibility, contraindications such as patients with pacemakers and cochlear implants, and, for some patients, claustrophobia. The magnetic pulses affect the electron spin, which produces signal variations that are displayed as an image.[56] MRI has the potential to directly visualize articular hyaline cartilage and can evaluate volume, thickness, morphology, and structural integrity.[57] MRI is sensitive and can show active inflammation in bone, soft tissues, and within the joint. Inflamed tissues, such as synovium and tenosynovium, contain inflammatory cells and increased vascularity with a higher water content (and therefore more H^+ ions) than normal tissue.[55] Bone damage can also be imaged with MRI. Erosions appear as breaks in cortical bone, whereas bone marrow edema is characterized by increased signal on fat-suppressed T2-weighted images.[55] Cartilage morphology (eg, area of thinning) can also be visualized with MRI.[55] Newer magnetic resonance (MR) techniques for assessing cartilage matrix can quantify cartilage integrity and may be a method to predict preclinical disease and progression. The ability to assess changes in water content[58] and proteoglycan density[59] along with specific cartilage pulse sequence protocols are helping to achieve a new understanding of cartilage biology.[57]

Evaluation of small joints requires high-resolution surface coils and newer gradient platforms. The OMERACT group has defined and validated an MRI scoring system for rheumatoid arthritis disease activity of the wrist and MCP joints called the Rheumatoid Arthritis Magnetic Resonance Imaging Score (RAMRIS). RAMRIS consists of a score for erosions, bone marrow edema, and synovitis as well as a composite score.[60] A limitation of RAMRIS is that scoring the study is time consuming and requires training for reproducible results.[61] Acquisition of MR images differs at various facilities. Use of contrast, magnet strength, and field of view (coned down, entire hand, both hands) all affect the sensitivity of the resultant image.[62–64] Efforts have been made to simplify the scoring of RAMRIS and to decrease invasiveness and the cost of MRI by eliminating the intravenous gadolinium. Ostergaard and colleagues[65] found that RAMRIS scores of bone erosions and bone edema did not change in studies without intravenous gadolinium, but synovitis scores were less reliable.

CAN MRI HELP PREDICT WHICH PATIENTS WITH UNDIFFERENTIATED INFLAMMATORY ARTHRITIS WILL DEVELOP RHEUMATOID ARTHRITIS?

An estimation of the risk of disease progression, joint damage, and loss of function are crucial to treatment decisions for patients who present with undifferentiated inflammatory arthritis. MRI evidence of bone edema and a combination of a distinct synovitis and erosion pattern are correlated with an increased risk of development of rheumatoid arthritis as defined by the 1987 American College of Radiology (ACR) criteria.[66] In patients with undifferentiated arthritis, bone edema on MRI predicts progression to rheumatoid arthritis both independently and when combined with positive rheumatoid factor or anti–cyclic citrullinated peptide antibodies.[67] MRI detection of synovitis and bone edema are also independent predictors of radiographic progression in patients with early rheumatoid arthritis.[68] McQueen and colleagues[69] showed that baseline bone edema predicted both JSN and the erosion component of the score, suggesting a influence on subchondral bone and cartilage. Biopsies of patients with late rheumatoid arthritis have shown that what is called bone edema on MRI represents inflammatory and vascular lymphoplasmacytic infiltrate of the bone marrow.[67]

Figs. 4 and **5** show how MRI and ultrasound can be used to diagnose early rheumatoid arthritis in patients with normal radiographs of the hands.

HOW OFTEN SHOULD PATIENTS HAVE IMAGING DONE AND WHICH IMAGING MODALITIES SHOULD BE USED?
Treat to Target

With advances in treatment and improved outcomes for many patients with rheumatoid arthritis, treat-to-target strategies have recently been developed for rheumatoid arthritis to improve patient care.[17,70] Treatment should be adjusted if the desired target is not rapidly reached, and the desired target should be sustained over time.[70] An international task force recommended in 2010 that the desired target should be based on validated clinical measures of remission or low disease activity, but that structural changes and functional impairment should be considered when making treatment decisions.[70] They recommended that radiographs be obtained annually and potential progression be estimated (not scored).[70] They noted the lag time of radiograph changes and the existence of other validated imaging modalities (ultrasound and MRI) but thought that scoring systems required further standardization and validation.[70] In 2011, the Canadian Rheumatology Association developed guidelines for the pharmacologic management of rheumatoid arthritis with traditional and biologic disease-modifying antirheumatic agents.[71] They recommended radiographs of the hands and feet as frequently as every 6 to 12 months in patients with recent-onset disease.[71] Radiographs could be performed at longer intervals for patients with established disease.[71] In addition, they recommended that change in

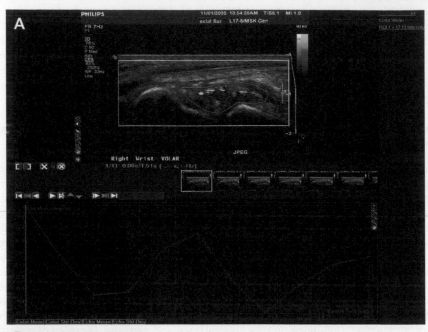

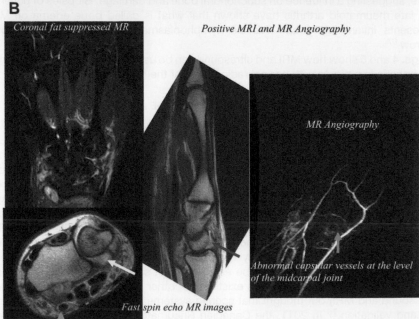

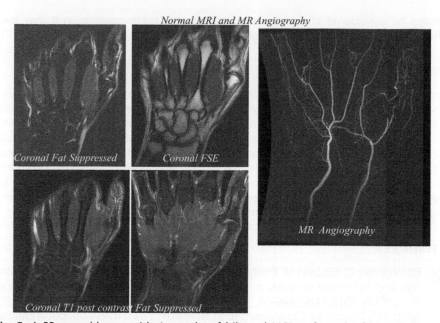

Fig. 5. A 33-year-old man with 4 months of bilateral MCP and proximal interphalangeal pain and swelling. He has minimal clinical synovitis, negative serologies, and a DAS of 2.61. Fat-suppressed and fast-spin echo MR show no evidence of synovitis affecting the wrist joints. MR angiography reveals no evidence of neovascularity. Coronal T1 fat-suppressed MR following injection of contrast also shows no abnormal areas of synovial enhancement in this normal study. (*From* Vasanth LC, Foo LF, Potter HG, et al. Using magnetic resonance angiography to measure abnormal synovial blood vessels in early inflammatory arthritis: a new imaging biomarker? J Rheumatol 2010;37(6):1133; with permission.)

Fig. 4. (*A*) A 23-year-old woman with 6 months of symmetric polyarthritis with morning stiffness. She had clinical synovitis, positive serologies, and a DAS of 5.32. Power Doppler ultrasound of the same patient shows the volar aspect of the wrist along the radioscaphoid joint. A region of interest encompasses hypoechoic soft tissue with increased vascularity. The graph plots the mean power Doppler signal intensity (dB/mm²) versus time. The pulsatility reflects the arterial component of the visualized vascularity. (*B*) Fat-suppressed coronal MRI shows a reactive bone marrow edema pattern affecting all joint compartments of the wrist. Axial and sagittal fast-spin echo MR images show synovial debris within the distended distal radioulnar (*yellow arrow*) and radiocarpal (*red arrow*) joints. Note also the presence of tenosynovitis of the flexor carpi radialis (*green arrow*). MR angiography shows the presence of new vessels (*blue arrow*) at the level of the midcarpal joint. (*From* Vasanth LC, Foo LF, Potter HG, et al. Using magnetic resonance angiography to measure abnormal synovial blood vessels in early inflammatory arthritis: a new imaging biomarker? J Rheumatol 2010;37(6):1133; with permission.)

therapy be considered in patients with radiographic progression even if they met criteria for low disease activity clinically.[71]

SUMMARY

Increased awareness of the need for early diagnosis of rheumatoid arthritis and advances in the ability to effectively treat rheumatoid arthritis have made disease remission and maintenance of function a reality for many patients. However, identification of patients with early inflammatory arthritis who are at risk for erosive disease remains a challenge. As more is learnt about risk factors for disease severity and the role of imaging techniques such as ultrasound and MRI is defined as a criterion for the diagnosis of early rheumatoid arthritis and treatment response, the ability to prevent disease progression in the form of joint damage and its attendant deformity and functional limitation will further improve.

REFERENCES

1. Bombardier C, Barbieri M, Parthan A, et al. The relationship between joint damage and functional disability in rheumatoid arthritis: a systematic review. Ann Rheum Dis 2012;71(6):836–44.
2. Bliddal H, Boesen M, Christensen R, et al. Imaging as a follow-up tool in clinical trials and clinical practice. Best Pract Res Clin Rheumatol 2008;22(6):1109–26.
3. Kassimos D, Creamer P. The hand X-ray in rheumatology. Hosp Med 2004;65(1): 13–7.
4. Hulsmans HM, Jacobs JW, van der Heijde DM, et al. The course of radiologic damage during the first six years of rheumatoid arthritis. Arthritis Rheum 2000;43(9):1927–40.
5. Drossaers-Bakker KW, Kroon HM, Zwinderman AH, et al. Radiographic damage of large joints in long-term rheumatoid arthritis and its relation to function. Rheumatology (Oxford) 2000;39(9):998–1003.
6. Ravindran V, Rachapalli S. An overview of commonly used radiographic scoring methods in rheumatoid arthritis clinical trials. Clin Rheumatol 2011;30(1):1–6.
7. Genant HK. Interleukin-1 receptor antagonist treatment of rheumatoid arthritis patients: radiologic progression and correlation of Genant/Sharp and Larsen scoring methods. Semin Arthritis Rheum 2001;30(5 Suppl 2):26–32.
8. van der Heijde DM. Assessment of radiographs in longitudinal observational studies. J Rheumatol Suppl 2004;69:46–7.
9. Ory PA. Interpreting radiographic data in rheumatoid arthritis. Ann Rheum Dis 2003;62(7):597–604.
10. van der Heijde D. How to read radiographs according to the Sharp/van der Heijde method. J Rheumatol 2000;27(1):261–3.
11. Dias EM, Lukas C, Landewe R, et al. Reliability and sensitivity to change of the Simple Erosion Narrowing Score compared with the Sharp-van der Heijde method for scoring radiographs in rheumatoid arthritis. Ann Rheum Dis 2008; 67(3):375–9.
12. van der Heijde D, Dankert T, Nieman F, et al. Reliability and sensitivity to change of a simplification of the Sharp/van der Heijde radiological assessment in rheumatoid arthritis. Rheumatology (Oxford) 1999;38(10):941–7.
13. Boers M, Verhoeven AC, Markusse HM, et al. Randomised comparison of combined step-down prednisolone, methotrexate and sulphasalazine with sulphasalazine alone in early rheumatoid arthritis. Lancet 1997;350(9074):309–18.

14. Genovese MC, Bathon JM, Martin RW, et al. Etanercept versus methotrexate in patients with early rheumatoid arthritis: two-year radiographic and clinical outcomes. Arthritis Rheum 2002;46(6):1443–50.
15. Grigor C, Capell H, Stirling A, et al. Effect of a treatment strategy of tight control for rheumatoid arthritis (the TICORA study): a single-blind randomised controlled trial. Lancet 2004;364(9430):263–9.
16. St Clair EW, van der Heijde DM, Smolen JS, et al. Combination of infliximab and methotrexate therapy for early rheumatoid arthritis: a randomized, controlled trial. Arthritis Rheum 2004;50(11):3432–43.
17. Goekoop-Ruiterman YP, de Vries-Bouwstra JK, Allaart CF, et al. Clinical and radiographic outcomes of four different treatment strategies in patients with early rheumatoid arthritis (the BeSt study): a randomized, controlled trial. Arthritis Rheum 2005;52(11):3381–90.
18. Siegert CE, Vleming LJ, Vandenbroucke JP, et al. Measurement of disability in Dutch rheumatoid arthritis patients. Clin Rheumatol 1984;3(3):305–9.
19. Breedveld FC, Weisman MH, Kavanaugh AF, et al. The PREMIER study: a multicenter, randomized, double-blind clinical trial of combination therapy with adalimumab plus methotrexate versus methotrexate alone or adalimumab alone in patients with early, aggressive rheumatoid arthritis who had not had previous methotrexate treatment. Arthritis Rheum 2006;54(1):26–37.
20. Emery P, Breedveld FC, Hall S, et al. Comparison of methotrexate monotherapy with a combination of methotrexate and etanercept in active, early, moderate to severe rheumatoid arthritis (COMET): a randomised, double-blind, parallel treatment trial. Lancet 2008;372(9636):375–82.
21. Keystone E, Heijde D, Mason D Jr, et al. Certolizumab pegol plus methotrexate is significantly more effective than placebo plus methotrexate in active rheumatoid arthritis: findings of a fifty-two-week, phase III, multicenter, randomized, double-blind, placebo-controlled, parallel-group study. Arthritis Rheum 2008; 58(11):3319–29.
22. Bruynesteyn K, van der Heijde D, Boers M, et al. Determination of the minimal clinically important difference in rheumatoid arthritis joint damage of the Sharp/van der Heijde and Larsen/Scott scoring methods by clinical experts and comparison with the smallest detectable difference. Arthritis Rheum 2002;46(4):913–20.
23. van der Heijde D, Landewe R, Klareskog L, et al. Presentation and analysis of data on radiographic outcome in clinical trials: experience from the TEMPO study. Arthritis Rheum 2005;52(1):49–60.
24. van der Heijde D, Simon L, Smolen J, et al. How to report radiographic data in randomized clinical trials in rheumatoid arthritis: guidelines from a roundtable discussion. Arthritis Rheum 2002;47(2):215–8.
25. Landewe R, van der Heijde D. Radiographic progression depicted by probability plots: presenting data with optimal use of individual values. Arthritis Rheum 2004;50(3):699–706.
26. Scott DL, Pugner K, Kaarela K, et al. The links between joint damage and disability in rheumatoid arthritis. Rheumatology (Oxford) 2000;39(2):122–32.
27. Smolen JS, Aletaha D, Grisar JC, et al. Estimation of a numerical value for joint damage-related physical disability in rheumatoid arthritis clinical trials. Ann Rheum Dis 2010;69(6):1058–64.
28. Rezaei H, Saevarsdottir S, Forslind K, et al. In early rheumatoid arthritis, patients with a good initial response to methotrexate have excellent 2-year clinical outcomes, but radiological progression is not fully prevented: data from the

methotrexate responders population in the SWEFOT trial. Ann Rheum Dis 2012; 71(2):186–91.

29. Landewe RB, Boers M, van der Heijde DM. How to interpret radiological progression in randomized clinical trials? Rheumatology (Oxford) 2003;42(1): 2–5.

30. Makinen H, Kautiainen H, Hannonen P, et al. Is DAS28 an appropriate tool to assess remission in rheumatoid arthritis? Ann Rheum Dis 2005;64(10):1410–3.

31. Aletaha D, Smolen JS. Joint damage in rheumatoid arthritis progresses in remission according to the Disease Activity Score in 28 joints and is driven by residual swollen joints. Arthritis Rheum 2011;63(12):3702–11.

32. Bathon JM, Martin RW, Fleischmann RM, et al. A comparison of etanercept and methotrexate in patients with early rheumatoid arthritis. N Engl J Med 2000; 343(22):1586–93.

33. Klareskog L, van der Heijde D, de Jager JP, et al. Therapeutic effect of the combination of etanercept and methotrexate compared with each treatment alone in patients with rheumatoid arthritis: double-blind randomised controlled trial. Lancet 2004;363(9410):675–81.

34. Smolen JS, Kalden JR, Scott DL, et al. Efficacy and safety of leflunomide compared with placebo and sulphasalazine in active rheumatoid arthritis: a double-blind, randomised, multicentre trial. European Leflunomide Study Group. Lancet 1999;353(9149):259–66.

35. Gandjbakhch F, Conaghan PG, Ejbjerg B, et al. Synovitis and osteitis are very frequent in rheumatoid arthritis clinical remission: results from an MRI study of 294 patients in clinical remission or low disease activity state. J Rheumatol 2011;38(9):2039–44.

36. Landewe R, van der Heijde D, Klareskog L, et al. Disconnect between inflammation and joint destruction after treatment with etanercept plus methotrexate: results from the trial of etanercept and methotrexate with radiographic and patient outcomes. Arthritis Rheum 2006;54(10):3119–25.

37. Smolen JS, Han C, Bala M, et al. Evidence of radiographic benefit of treatment with infliximab plus methotrexate in rheumatoid arthritis patients who had no clinical improvement: a detailed subanalysis of data from the anti-tumor necrosis factor trial in rheumatoid arthritis with concomitant therapy study. Arthritis Rheum 2005;52(4):1020–30.

38. Boers M, van Tuyl L, van den Broek M, et al. Meta-analysis suggests that intensive non-biological combination therapy with step-down prednisolone (COBRA strategy) may also 'disconnect' disease activity and damage in rheumatoid arthritis. Ann Rheum Dis 2013;72(3):406–9.

39. Smolen JS, Avila JC, Aletaha D. Tocilizumab inhibits progression of joint damage in rheumatoid arthritis irrespective of its anti-inflammatory effects: disassociation of the link between inflammation and destruction. Ann Rheum Dis 2012; 71(5):687–93.

40. Keystone E. Recent concepts in the inhibition of radiographic progression with biologics. Curr Opin Rheumatol 2009;21(3):231–7.

41. Lillegraven S, Prince FH, Shadick NA, et al. Remission and radiographic outcome in rheumatoid arthritis: application of the 2011 ACR/EULAR remission criteria in an observational cohort. Ann Rheum Dis 2012;71(5):681–6.

42. Lipsky PE, van der Heijde DM, St Clair EW, et al. Infliximab and methotrexate in the treatment of rheumatoid arthritis. Anti-Tumor Necrosis Factor Trial in Rheumatoid Arthritis with Concomitant Therapy Study Group. N Engl J Med 2000; 343(22):1594–602.

43. McQueen FM, Benton N, Crabbe J, et al. What is the fate of erosions in early rheumatoid arthritis? Tracking individual lesions using x rays and magnetic resonance imaging over the first two years of disease. Ann Rheum Dis 2001;60(9): 859–68.
44. Rau R, Wassenberg S, Herborn G, et al. Identification of radiologic healing phenomena in patients with rheumatoid arthritis. J Rheumatol 2001;28(12):2608–15.
45. Sharp JT, Van Der Heijde D, Boers M, et al. Repair of erosions in rheumatoid arthritis does occur. Results from 2 studies by the OMERACT Subcommittee on Healing of Erosions. J Rheumatol 2003;30(5):1102–7.
46. Ostergaard M, Pedersen SJ, Dohn UM. Imaging in rheumatoid arthritis–status and recent advances for magnetic resonance imaging, ultrasonography, computed tomography and conventional radiography. Best Pract Res Clin Rheumatol 2008;22(6):1019–44.
47. Baillet A, Gaujoux-Viala C, Mouterde G, et al. Comparison of the efficacy of sonography, magnetic resonance imaging and conventional radiography for the detection of bone erosions in rheumatoid arthritis patients: a systematic review and meta-analysis. Rheumatology (Oxford) 2011;50(6):1137–47.
48. Ohrndorf S, Backhaus M. Advances in sonographic scoring of rheumatoid arthritis. Ann Rheum Dis 2013;72(Suppl 2):ii69–75.
49. Szkudlarek M, Court-Payen M, Jacobsen S, et al. Interobserver agreement in ultrasonography of the finger and toe joints in rheumatoid arthritis. Arthritis Rheum 2003;48(4):955–62.
50. Wakefield RJ, D'Agostino MA, Iagnocco A, et al. The OMERACT Ultrasound Group: status of current activities and research directions. J Rheumatol 2007; 34(4):848–51.
51. Grassi W, Lamanna G, Farina A, et al. Sonographic imaging of normal and osteoarthritic cartilage. Semin Arthritis Rheum 1999;28(6):398–403.
52. McQueen FM, Ostergaard M. Established rheumatoid arthritis – new imaging modalities. Best Pract Res Clin Rheumatol 2007;21(5):841–56.
53. Kazam JK, Nazarian LN, Miller TT, et al. Sonographic evaluation of femoral trochlear cartilage in patients with knee pain. J Ultrasound Med 2011;30(6): 797–802.
54. Naredo E, Collado P, Cruz A, et al. Longitudinal power Doppler ultrasonographic assessment of joint inflammatory activity in early rheumatoid arthritis: predictive value in disease activity and radiologic progression. Arthritis Rheum 2007;57(1): 116–24.
55. McQueen FM. The use of MRI in early RA. Rheumatology (Oxford) 2008;47(11): 1597–9.
56. Peterfy CG. Magnetic resonance imaging of the wrist in rheumatoid arthritis. Semin Musculoskelet Radiol 2001;5(3):275–88.
57. Wang Y, Wluka AE, Jones G, et al. Use magnetic resonance imaging to assess articular cartilage. Ther Adv Musculoskelet Dis 2012;4(2):77–97.
58. Liess C, Lusse S, Karger N, et al. Detection of changes in cartilage water content using MRI T2-mapping in vivo. Osteoarthritis Cartilage 2002;10(12):907–13.
59. Akella SV, Regatte RR, Gougoutas AJ, et al. Proteoglycan-induced changes in T1rho-relaxation of articular cartilage at 4T. Magn Reson Med 2001;46(3): 419–23.
60. Ostergaard M, Peterfy C, Conaghan P, et al. OMERACT Rheumatoid Arthritis Magnetic Resonance Imaging Studies. Core set of MRI acquisitions, joint pathology definitions, and the OMERACT RA-MRI scoring system. J Rheumatol 2003;30(6):1385–6.

61. Ostergaard M, Edmonds J, McQueen F, et al. An introduction to the EULAR-OMERACT rheumatoid arthritis MRI reference image atlas. Ann Rheum Dis 2005;64(Suppl 1):i3–7.
62. Hodgson RJ, O'Connor PJ, Ridgway JP. Optimizing MRI for imaging peripheral arthritis. Semin Musculoskelet Radiol 2012;16(5):367–76.
63. Weckbach S. Whole-body MRI for inflammatory arthritis and other multifocal rheumatoid diseases. Semin Musculoskelet Radiol 2012;16(5):377–88.
64. Appel H, Hermann KG, Althoff CE, et al. Whole-body magnetic resonance imaging evaluation of widespread inflammatory lesions in a patient with ankylosing spondylitis before and after 1 year of treatment with infliximab. J Rheumatol 2007;34(12):2497–8.
65. Ostergaard M, Conaghan PG, O'Connor P, et al. Reducing invasiveness, duration, and cost of magnetic resonance imaging in rheumatoid arthritis by omitting intravenous contrast injection – Does it change the assessment of inflammatory and destructive joint changes by the OMERACT RAMRIS? J Rheumatol 2009; 36(8):1806–10.
66. Machado PM, Koevoets R, Bombardier C, et al. The value of magnetic resonance imaging and ultrasound in undifferentiated arthritis: a systematic review. J Rheumatol Suppl 2011;87:31–7.
67. McQueen FM. Bone marrow edema and osteitis in rheumatoid arthritis: the imaging perspective. Arthritis Res Ther 2012;14(5):224.
68. Boyesen P, Haavardsholm EA, Ostergaard M, et al. MRI in early rheumatoid arthritis: synovitis and bone marrow oedema are independent predictors of subsequent radiographic progression. Ann Rheum Dis 2011;70(3):428–33.
69. McQueen FM, Benton N, Perry D, et al. Bone edema scored on magnetic resonance imaging scans of the dominant carpus at presentation predicts radiographic joint damage of the hands and feet six years later in patients with rheumatoid arthritis. Arthritis Rheum 2003;48(7):1814–27.
70. Smolen JS, Aletaha D, Bijlsma JW, et al. Treating rheumatoid arthritis to target: recommendations of an international task force. Ann Rheum Dis 2010;69(4): 631–7.
71. Bykerk VP, Akhavan P, Hazlewood GS, et al. Canadian Rheumatology Association recommendations for pharmacological management of rheumatoid arthritis with traditional and biologic disease-modifying antirheumatic drugs. J Rheumatol 2012;39(8):1559–82.

Osteoarthritis
A Review of Strengths and Weaknesses of Different Imaging Options

Ali Guermazi, MD, PhD[a],*, Daichi Hayashi, MD, PhD[a],
Frank W. Roemer, MD[a], David T. Felson, MD, MPH[b]

KEYWORDS

- Osteoarthritis • Imaging • Radiography • MR imaging • Ultrasonography • CT
- PET

KEY POINTS

- Radiography is still the most widely used imaging modality for clinical management of patients with osteoarthritis.
- A reduction in the loss of joint space width represents the only end point recommended by the US Food and Drug Administration for structural disease progression in clinical trials.
- Because magnetic resonance (MR) imaging visualizes many structures within the knee and directly visualizes cartilage, it has a unique role in exploring the natural history of osteoarthritis and in the search for new therapies.
- The main MR imaging-based assessment approaches for osteoarthritis are semiquantitative, quantitative, and compositional.
- Ultrasonography may be useful to evaluate synovial disease in osteoarthritis, particularly in the hand.

RADIOGRAPHY

This review article focuses on osteoarthritis (OA) of the knee joint to summarize the current role and limitations of each imaging modality. The first modality to be

Role of the Funding Source: No funding received.

Competing Interests: Dr Guermazi has received consultancies, speaking fees, or honoraria from Genzyme, Stryker, Merck Serono, Novartis and Astra Zeneca and is the President of Boston Imaging Core Laboratory (BICL), a company providing image assessment services. He received a research grant from General Electric Healthcare. Dr Roemer is Chief Medical Officer and shareholder of BICL. Dr Roemer has received consultancies, speaking fees, or honoraria from Merck Serono and the National Institutes of Health.

[a] Department of Radiology, Boston University School of Medicine, 820 Harrison Avenue, FGH Building, 3rd Floor, Boston, MA 02118, USA; [b] Clinical Epidemiology Research and Training Unit, Boston University School of Medicine, 650 Albany Street, Suite X200, Boston, MA 02118, USA

* Corresponding author.

E-mail address: guermazi@bu.edu

Rheum Dis Clin N Am 39 (2013) 567–591

http://dx.doi.org/10.1016/j.rdc.2013.02.001

described is radiography, which is the simplest, least expensive, and most widely used. It enables detection of OA-associated bony features such as osteophytes, subchondral sclerosis, and cysts (**Fig. 1**).[1] Radiography can also determine joint space width (JSW), which is a surrogate for cartilage thickness and meniscal integrity in knees, but precise measurement of each of these articular structures is not possible with conventional radiograph-based methods.[2] Despite this limitation, slowing of radiographically detected joint space narrowing (JSN) is the only structural end point approved by the US Food and Drug Administration (FDA) to show efficacy of disease-modifying OA drugs in phase 3 clinical trials. OA is radiographically defined by the presence of marginal osteophytes.[3] Progression of JSN is the most commonly used criterion for the assessment of structural OA progression, and the total loss of JSW (bone-on-bone appearance) is one of the indicators for joint replacement.

Recent research efforts have revealed that cartilage loss is not the sole contributor to joint space loss but that changes in the meniscus such as meniscal extrusion also contribute to JSN (**Fig. 2**).[2] The lack of sensitivity and specificity of radiography for the detection of OA-associated articular tissue damage, and its poor sensitivity to change at follow-up imaging, are other important limitations of radiography. Variations in knee positioning, which occur during image acquisition despite standardization, can also be problematic. Such variations can affect the quantitative measurement of various radiographic parameters, including JSW.[4] Despite these limitations, radiography remains the gold standard for establishing an imaging-based diagnosis of OA and for assessment of structural modification in clinical trials of knee OA.

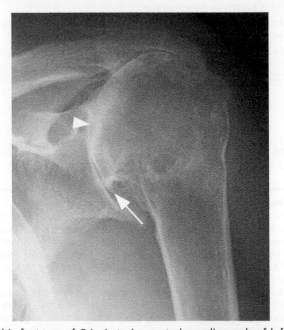

Fig. 1. Radiographic features of OA. Anterior-posterior radiograph of left shoulder shows severe glenohumeral OA caused by rotator cuff arthropathy. Note the complete loss of subacromial joint space and neoarticulation between the superior humeral head and acromion because of a long-standing complete tear of the supraspinatus tendon with retraction (not visualized by radiograph). Characteristic signs of advanced radiographic OA include subchondral sclerosis (*arrowhead*) and inferior humeral osteophytes (*arrow*).

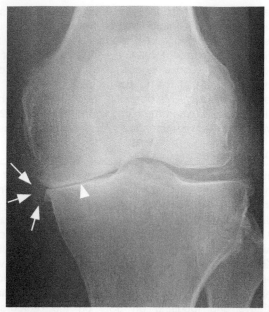

Fig. 2. Radiographic JSN. Severe knee OA as visualized by radiography. Anterior-posterior radiograph shows complete loss of medial tibiofemoral joint space (*arrowhead*). JSN is a result of cartilage damage and meniscal disease, including extrusion as seen in this example. The calcified body of the medial meniscus is markedly extruded medially, which contributes to joint space loss (*arrows*).

Semiquantitative Assessments

The severity of radiographic OA can be assessed with semiquantitative scoring systems. The Kellgren and Lawrence (KL) grading system[5] is a widely accepted scheme for defining radiographic OA based on the presence of a definite osteophyte (= grade 2). However, KL grading has its limitations; in particular, KL grade 3 includes all degrees of definite JSN, regardless of the extent. Modification of KL grading has been suggested to increase sensitivity to change in longitudinal knee OA studies,[6] with a recommendation that OA be defined by a combination of JSN and the presence of definite osteophytes in a knee that did not have this combination on the previous radiographic assessment. For OA progression, a focus on JSN alone using either a semiquantitative[7] or a quantitative approach was recommended.

The Osteoarthritis Research Society International (OARSI) atlas[1] provides grades for specific features of OA rather than global scores like the KL scheme. The atlas grades tibiofemoral JSW and osteophytes separately for each compartment of the knee (medial tibiofemoral, lateral tibiofemoral, and patellofemoral). A recent study using data from the OA Initiative and the OARSI atlas for semiquantitative grading of JSN showed that centralized radiographic reading is important from the point of observer reliability, because even expert readers seem to apply different thresholds for JSN grading.[8]

Quantitative Assessments

JSW is the distance between the projected femoral and tibial margins on the radiographic image. Measurement is manual or with software and the measurement is called quantitative JSW. Quantification using image-processing software requires a digital image, whether digitized plain films or images acquired using fully digital modalities such as computed radiography and digital radiography. Minimum JSW is the standard metric, but some groups have investigated the use of location-specific JSW.[9-11] Various degrees of responsiveness have been observed depending on the degree of OA severity, length of the follow-up period, and the knee-positioning protocol.[11,12] Measurements of JSW obtained from knee radiographs have been found to be reliable, especially when the study lasted longer than 2 years and when the radiographs were obtained with the knee in a standardized flexed position.[13]

Recent Research Developments

Radiography still has a role to play in OA trials because of its lower cost and greater accessibility compared with magnetic resonance (MR) imaging. Duryea and colleagues[12] reported that measures of location-specific JSW, using software analysis of digital knee radiographic images, were comparable with MR imaging in detecting OA progression. A clinical trial by Mazzuca and colleagues[14] showed that varus malalignment of the lower limb negated the slowing of structural progression of medial JSN by doxycycline. Kinds and colleagues[15] showed that, in patients with knee pain at baseline, measurement of osteophyte area and minimum JSW predicted radiographic OA occurring 5 years later. Using data from the Multicenter Osteoarthritis Study and Osteoarthritis Initiative and focusing on JSN on the radiograph, Felson and colleagues[16] showed that valgus malalignment of the lower limb increases the risk of disease progression in knees with radiographic lateral knee OA. Even in knees without radiographic knee OA, valgus alignment more than 3° was associated with incident radiographic lateral knee OA at follow-up.

Two older methods (bone texture analysis and tomosynthesis) have experienced a revival lately. Bone texture analysis extracts from conventional radiographs information on two-dimensional trabecular bone texture that relates directly to three-dimensional bone structure. Woloszynski and colleagues[17] showed that bone texture may be a predictor of progression of tibiofemoral OA. Tomosynthesis generates an arbitrary number of section images from a single pass of the radiograph tube. Hayashi and colleagues[18] showed that tomosynthesis is more sensitive in the detection of osteophytes and subchondral cysts than radiography, using 3T MR imaging as the reference.

MR IMAGING

Because of the high cost per examination, MR imaging is not routinely used in clinical management of patients with OA. However, MR has become a key imaging tool for OA research[19-21] because of its ability to visualize disease in structures not imaged by radiography (ie, articular cartilage, menisci, ligaments, synovium, capsular structures, fluid collections and bone marrow) (**Fig. 3**).[22-33] With MR imaging, the joint can be evaluated as a whole organ; multiple tissue changes can be monitored simultaneously over several time points; pathologic changes of preradiographic OA can be detected at an earlier stage of the disease; and physiologic changes within joint tissues (eg, cartilage and menisci) can be assessed before morphologic changes become apparent (**Fig. 4**). MR imaging has helped OA investigators to move away from the traditional notion that the OA is an isolated disease of articular cartilage. Contemporary models recognize the involvement of the entire synovial joint organ and view OA as the clinical and pathologic outcome of a range of disorders that results in structural and functional failure of the synovial joint organ with loss and erosion of cartilage, subchondral bone alteration, meniscal damage, synovitis, and overgrowth of bone

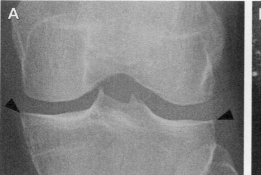
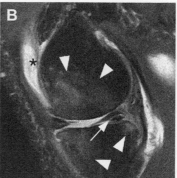

Fig. 3. Multitissue visualization of degenerative joint disease by MR imaging. (*A*) Anterior-posterior radiograph shows small medial and lateral tibial osteophytes (*arrowheads*) and no JSN. No additional features of OA are seen. (*B*) Sagittal intermediate-weighted fat-saturated MR image of the same joint depicts multiple joint pathologies not appreciated on the radiograph: a horizontal-oblique degenerative tear of the posterior horn of the medial meniscus (*arrow*), several tibial and femoral bone marrow lesions (*arrowheads*), and marked effusion synovitis (*asterisk*).

(osteophytes).[34] Nonetheless, radiologic-surgical correlation studies have shown that direct visualization of joint tissues by arthroscopy is more accurate in diagnosing cartilage loss and meniscal and ligamentous damages,[35–37] and thus in the clinical setting, arthroscopic examination remains the gold standard investigation before definitive treatment planning.[37]

It is necessary to select appropriate MR pulse sequences for the purpose of each study (**Fig. 5**). For example, focal cartilage defects and bone marrow lesions are best assessed using fluid-sensitive fast spin-echo sequences (eg, T2-weighted, proton density-weighted, or intermediate-weighted) with fat suppression (**Fig. 6**).[21,25] Moreover, MR images may sometimes be affected by artifacts that mimic

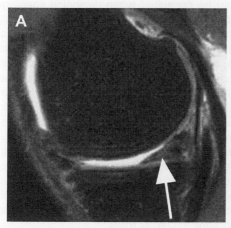
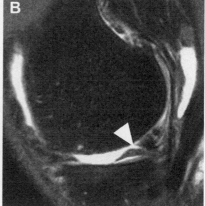

Fig. 4. Sensitivity of MR imaging to early joint disease. Example of the development of a meniscal tear over 2 years. (*A*) Baseline sagittal intermediate-weighted fat-saturated image shows intrameniscal signal changes of the medial posterior horn consistent with mucoid degeneration (*arrow*). (*B*) Follow-up image 2 years later depicts an incident oblique tear of the posterior horn reaching the meniscal upper surface (*arrowhead*).

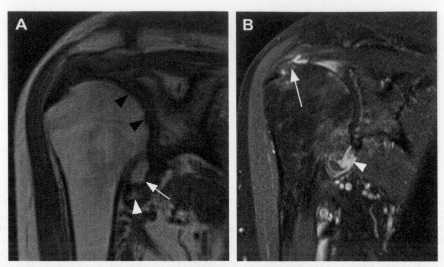

Fig. 5. Relevance of sequence selection for visualization of different OA features. (*A*) Coronal nonfat-suppressed T1-weighted image of glenohumeral OA. Bony disease is well visualized on this T1-weighted nonfat-suppressed MR image. A large inferior osteophyte is present at the humeral head (*arrow*) and small calcified loose body is adjacent to the osteophyte (*white arrowhead*). Subchondral sclerosis is depicted as linear hypointensity directly adjacent to the humeral cortex (*black arrowheads*). (*B*) Coronal T1-weighted fat-saturated image after intravenous contrast administration shows marked synovitis in the axillary recess (*arrowhead*). In addition, there is a complete tear of the supraspinatus tendon medial to the tendon attachment at the greater tubercle (*arrow*).

pathologic findings. For example, susceptibility artifacts can be misinterpreted as cartilage loss or meniscal tear if the observer is unaware of the phenomenon (**Fig. 7**). Gradient recalled echo sequences are known to be particularly prone to this type of artifact.[38] To ascertain optimal assessment of MR imaging-derived data, trained musculoskeletal radiologists should be consulted when designing imaging-based OA studies or when interpreting data from the studies.

An MR imaging-based definition of OA has recently been proposed.[39] Tibiofemoral OA on MR imaging is defined as either (1) the presence of both definite osteophyte formation and full-thickness cartilage loss, or (2) the presence of 1 of the features in (1) and 1 of the following: subchondral bone marrow lesion or cyst not associated with meniscal or ligamentous attachments; meniscal subluxation, maceration, or degenerative (horizontal) tear; partial thickness cartilage loss; and bone attrition. In addition, with MR imaging, OA can be classified into hypertrophic and atrophic phenotypes, according to the size of osteophytes.[40]

The use of MR imaging has led to significant findings about the association of pain with bone marrow lesions[41,42] and synovitis,[43] with implications for future OA clinical trials. Systematic reviews have shown that MR imaging biomarkers in OA have concurrent and predictive validity, with good responsiveness and reliability.[44,45] The OARSI-FDA working group now recommends MR imaging as a suitable imaging tool for the assessment of cartilage morphology in clinical trials.[19]

Semiquantitative MR Imaging Scoring Systems for Knee OA

A detailed review of semiquantitative MR imaging assessment of OA has been published recently,[46] and this approach is summarized in this article. In addition to the

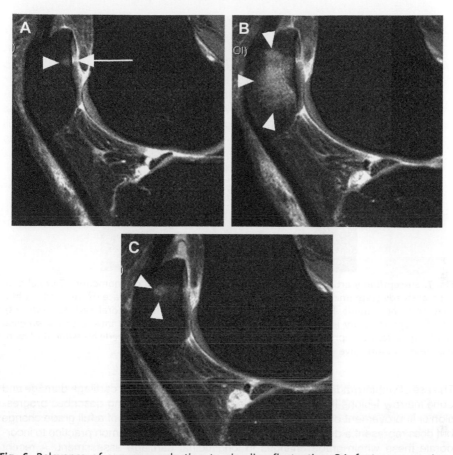

Fig. 6. Relevance of sequence selection to visualize fluctuating OA features over time. (*A*) Sagittal intermediate fat-saturated MR image shows small full-thickness focal cartilage defect (*arrow*) and a small adjacent subchondral bone marrow lesion (*arrowhead*). (*B*) At 12-month follow-up, there is a marked increase in the bone marrow lesion (*arrowheads*), whereas the cartilage defect remains unchanged in size. (*C*) At 24-month follow-up, there is a marked regression of the bone marrow lesion (*arrowheads*), whereas the cartilage defect remains unchanged. Bone marrow lesions are depicted to their full extent only on standard fat-suppressed turbo spin-echo sequences.

3 well-established scoring systems (the Whole Organ Magnetic Resonance Imaging Score [WORMS],[47] the Knee Osteoarthritis Scoring System,[48] and the Boston Leeds Osteoarthritis Knee Score [BLOKS][49]), a new scoring system called the MR Imaging Osteoarthritis Knee Score (MOAKS)[50] has been added to the literature. Of the 3 systems, WORMS and BLOKS have been widely disseminated and used, although only a few studies have directly compared the 2 systems. Two recent studies identified the relative strengths and weaknesses of the 2 systems in regard to certain features assumed to be most relevant to the natural history of the disease, including cartilage, meniscus, and bone marrow lesions.[51,52] WORMS and BLOKS both have weaknesses, and it may be difficult to decide which is more suitable for a particular study. In addition, both of these systems have undergone unpublished modifications, and their application in a particular study may vary markedly from the original description.

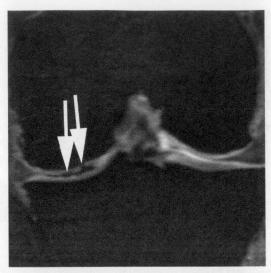

Fig. 7. Susceptibility artifacts caused by intra-articular vacuum phenomenon. Coronal dual echo at steady state image shows a hypointense line in the joint space of the medial tibio-femoral compartment. Hypointensity signal extends into the femoral cartilage (*arrows*). Usually hyperintensity is seen within the joint space, representing intra-articular synovial fluid. Hypointensity represents a vacuum phenomenon and may impede assessment of cartilage using quantitative or semiquantitative measures.

The use of within-grade changes for longitudinal assessment of cartilage damage and bone marrow lesions is a good example.[53] Within-grade scoring describes progression or improvement of a lesion that does not meet the criteria of a full grade change but does represent a definite visual change. It has become common practice to incorporate these within-grade changes in longitudinal cartilage assessment. A recent study showed that within-grade changes in semiquantitative MR imaging assessment of cartilage and bone marrow lesions are valid and their use may increase the sensitivity of semiquantitative readings for detecting longitudinal changes in these structures.[53]

By integrating expert readers' experience with all of the available scoring tools and the published data comparing different scoring systems, MOAKS provides a refined scoring tool for cross-sectional and longitudinal semiquantitative MR assessment of knee OA (**Fig. 8**). It includes semiquantitative scoring of pathologic features: bone marrow lesions; subchondral cysts; articular cartilage; osteophytes; Hoffa synovitis and synovitis-effusion; meniscus; tendons, and ligaments; and periarticular features such as cysts and bursitides. Using MOAKS, Bloecker and colleagues[54] showed that knees with medial JSN are associated with greater meniscal extrusion and damage compared with knees without medial JSN. MOAKS is a new scoring system, and more data are needed to show its validity and reliability in OA studies.

Synovitis is an important feature of OA and is associated with pain.[43,55] Although synovitis can be evaluated with noncontrast-enhanced MR imaging by using the presence of signal changes in the Hoffa fat pad or joint effusion as an indirect marker of synovitis, only contrast-enhanced MR imaging can reveal the true extent of synovial inflammation (**Fig. 9**).[56] Scoring systems of synovitis based on contrast-enhanced MR imaging have been published,[43,55] and these could be used in clinical trials of new OA drugs that target synovitis.

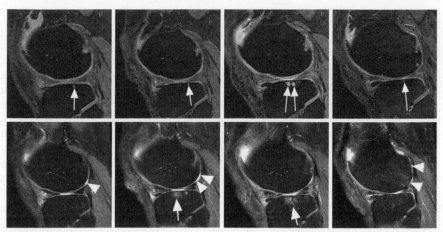

Fig. 8. Longitudinal assessment of knee OA over 3 years by MR imaging. Left column depicts baseline images; the other columns show (*left to right*) follow-up at 1 year, 2 years, and 3 years. Images in the upper row are dual echo at steady state (DESS) images, and those in the lower row are intermediate-weighted fat-saturated images of the same slice position acquired at the same visit. The baseline intermediate-weighted fat-saturated image at the bottom left shows a focal full-thickness cartilage defect of the posterior femoral condyle (*arrowhead*) that is not visible on the sagittal DESS image, a high-resolution three-dimensional gradient echo sequence (*far left, upper row*). The superiority of conventional spin-echo sequences for focal defects is a result of the superior contrast between joint fluid and cartilage surface causing an arthrographic effect. In the second column, the bottom intermediate-weighted fat-saturated image clearly depicts an increase in defect size (*arrow-heads*). At the 24-month visit (*third column*), there is further increase in cartilage damage at the posterior lateral femur, which is superiorly depicted on the intermediate-weighted fat-saturated image. At the 36-month visit (*bottom right*), there is further increase in cartilage damage (*arrowheads*). Note also the fluctuation of the tibial bone marrow lesion with no lesion at the baseline, a moderate-sized ill-defined lesion at 12 months (*arrow*), increase in size (*arrow*), and development of a cystic part within that same lesion at 24 months, and marked regression at the 36-month visit. DESS images in the upper row are sensitive to visualization of the cystic part of bone marrow lesions (*arrows*) but cannot depict the ill-defined nature of lesions.

Semiquantitative MR Imaging Scoring System for Hand OA

Radiography is still the imaging modality of choice clinically for OA of the hand, but the use of more sensitive imaging techniques such as ultrasonography and MR imaging is becoming more common, especially in OA research (**Fig. 10**). However, the literature concerning MR imaging of pathologic features of hand OA is still sparse, and studies have been performed without applying standardized methods.[57,58] In 2011, Haugen and colleagues[59] proposed a semiquantitative MR imaging scoring system for hand OA features using an extremity 1.0-T MR system, called the Oslo Hand OA MRI Score. The system incorporates osteophyte presence and JSN (0–3 scale) and malalignment (absence/presence) in analogue to the OARSI atlas.[1] Scoring of key pathologic features such as synovitis, flexor tenosynovitis, erosions, osteophytes, JSN, and bone marrow lesions showed good to very good intrareader and interreader reliability. Using this scoring system, Haugen and colleagues[60] showed that MR imaging could detect approximately twice as many joints with erosions and osteophytes as conventional radiography (*P*<.001), but identification of JSN, cysts, and malalignment was

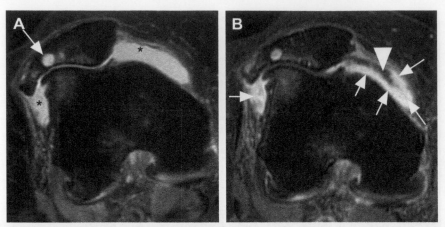

Fig. 9. Visualization of synovitis using nonenhanced and contrast-enhanced MR imaging. (*A*) Axial proton density-weighted fat-saturated image shows marked hyperintensity within the joint cavity, suggesting severe joint effusion (*asterisks*). In addition, there is a large sub-chondral cyst in the lateral facet of the patella. (*B*) Axial T1-weighted fat-saturated image after contrast administration clearly shows severe synovial thickening depicted as contrast enhancement (*arrows*). Arrowhead points to true amount of effusion, which is discrete and visualized as linear hypointensity only within the joint cavity.

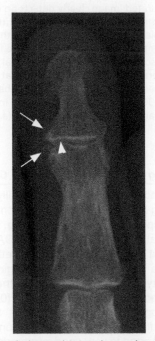

Fig. 10. Finger OA. Distal interphalangeal joint shows characteristic radiographic signs of OA, including marginal osteophyte formation (*arrows*) and asymmetric JSN (*arrowhead*). Soft tissue changes such as synovitis are only poorly visualized by radiograph and are depicted as increased soft tissue opacity, reflecting soft tissue swelling.

similar. The same group of investigators in another study showed that MR imaging-assessed moderate/severe synovitis, bone marrow lesions, erosions, attrition, and osteophytes were associated with joint tenderness independently of each other.[61] These studies showed that some of the semiquantitatively assessed MR imaging features of hand OA may be potential targets for therapeutic interventions.

Semiquantitative MR Imaging Scoring System for Hip OA

The hip joint has a spherical structure and its thin covering of articular hyaline cartilage makes MR imaging assessment of the hip more difficult than the knee. Roemer and colleagues[62] developed a whole-organ semiquantitative multifeature scoring method called the Hip Osteoarthritis MRI Scoring System (HOAMS) for use in observational studies and clinical trials of hip joints. In HOAMS, 14 articular features are assessed: cartilage morphology, subchondral bone marrow lesions, subchondral cysts, osteophytes, acetabular labrum, synovitis (scored only when contrast-enhanced sequences are available), joint effusion, loose bodies, attrition, dysplasia, trochanteric bursitis/insertional tendonitis of the greater trochanter, labral hypertrophy, paralabral cysts, and herniation pits at the superolateral femoral neck. HOAMS showed satisfactory reliability and good agreement concerning intraobserver and interobserver assessment, but further validation, assessment of responsiveness, and iterative refinement are still needed to maximize its usefulness in clinical trials and epidemiologic studies.

Quantitative Analysis of Articular Cartilage and Other Tissues

Quantitative measurement of cartilage morphology segments the cartilage image and exploits the three-dimensional nature of MR imaging data sets to evaluate tissue dimensions (such as thickness and volume) or signal as continuous variables. Examples of nomenclature for MR imaging-based cartilage measures were proposed by Eckstein and colleagues[63]: VC = cartilage volume; tAB = total area of subchondral bone; dAB = denuded area of subchondral bone, ThCtAB.Me = mean cartilage thickness over the tAB. Because many of these measures are strongly related, Buck and colleagues[64] identified an efficient subset of core measures (tAB, and dAB) that can provide a comprehensive description of cartilage morphology and its longitudinal changes, in knees with or without OA. The same group also proposed strategies (the ordered values approach and the extended ordered values approach) for more efficiently analyzing longitudinal changes in (subregional) cartilage thickness.[65,66] Not all knees lose cartilage in the same region, and these analytical methods track the region that is losing the most cartilage in each knee independently of anatomic location. This approach improves discrimination between different types of study participants (eg, those with or without radiographic knee OA).

Quantitative cartilage morphometry has been applied in various OA studies.[67–70] Quantitative measures of articular cartilage structure, such as cartilage thickness loss and denuded areas of subchondral bone, have been shown to predict an important clinical outcome (ie, knee replacement).[70] However, investigators intending to use the quantitative morphometry approach in a multicenter study should be aware that data collected from different segmentation teams should be pooled only when equivalence is shown for the cartilage metrics of interest; Schneider and colleagues[71] showed that segmentation team differences dominated measurement variability in most cartilage regions for all image series.

Several investigators[72–74] have reported studies using MR imaging to quantitatively evaluate the menisci. Wirth and colleagues[72] presented a technique for three-dimensional and quantitative analysis of meniscal shape and position, which was shown to display adequate interobserver precision.[73] When examining healthy reference individuals using these techniques, the investigators reported that meniscus surface area strongly corresponds with (ipsilateral) tibial plateau area across both sexes and that tibial coverage by the meniscus is similar between men and women. However, for menisci, the location and presence of damage may have more clinical and biological meaning than how large the meniscus is. Other than menisci, investigators have used quantitative MR imaging to assess bone marrow lesions,[75] synovitis,[76] and joint effusion.[77] However, using segmentation approaches for ill-defined lesions such as bone marrow lesions is more challenging than segmentation of clearly delineated structures such as cartilage, menisci, and effusion.

Compositional MR Imaging

Compositional MR imaging allows visualization of the biochemical properties of different joint tissues. It may be sensitive to early, premorphologic changes that cannot be seen on conventional MR imaging. Most studies applying compositional MR imaging have focused on cartilage, although the technique can also be used to assess other tissues, such as the menisci or ligaments. Compositional imaging of cartilage matrix changes can be performed using advanced MR imaging techniques, such as delayed gadolinium-enhanced MR imaging of cartilage (dGEMRIC), T1 ρ, and T2 mapping **(Fig. 11)**.[78,79] Of these techniques, the first 2 take advantage of the concentration of highly negatively charged glycosaminoglycans (GAGs) in healthy hyaline cartilage; loss of these GAGs in focal areas affected by possible early disease can be visualized. Both dGEMRIC and T1 ρ focus on charge density in cartilage. In contrast, T2 concentrations are affected by a complex combination of collagen orientation and hydration of cartilage.

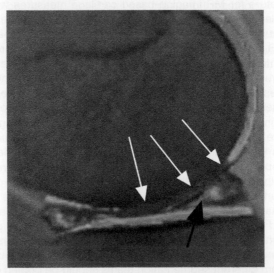

Fig. 11. Compositional MR image. Sagittal three-dimensional inversion recovery–prepared spoiled-gradient echo sequences were acquired 90 minutes after intravenous administration of gadolinium-diethylenetriamine penta-acetate^{2-}) for dGEMRIC assessment. Image shows decrease in the dGEMRIC index in the weight-bearing part of the medial femoral cartilage coded in red (*white arrows*), and the articular surface morphology remains intact. In addition, partial maceration of the posterior horn of the medial meniscus is observed (*black arrow*), which is likely responsible for biomechanical alterations leading to early cartilage damage.

Compositional MR imaging techniques are not routine in clinical practice and remain research tools that are available only at a limited number of institutions. Nevertheless, they have been applied in clinical trials and observational studies. In 2005, Roos and Dahlberg[80] used dGEMRIC in a randomized controlled trial involving 30 patients to visualize premorphologic changes of cartilage and showed that moderate exercise may improve the knee cartilage GAG content in patients at high risk of developing knee OA. More recently, in a placebo-controlled double-blind pilot study of collagen hydrolysate for mild knee OA, McAlindon and colleagues[81] reported that the dGEMRIC score increased (meaning higher GAG content and better cartilage status) in tibial cartilage regions of interest in patients receiving collagen hydrolysate and decreased in the placebo group. A significant difference was observed at 24 weeks. It will be interesting to see if macroscopic cartilage changes are associated with those early dGEMRIC findings in future studies. Van Gickel and colleagues[82] showed an increase in dGEMRIC indices of knee cartilage (meaning better cartilage status) in asymptomatic untrained women who were enrolled in a 10-week running program, when compared with sedentary controls. Souza and colleagues[83] reported that acute loading of the knee joint resulted in a significant decrease in T1 ρ and T2 relaxation times of the medial tibiofemoral compartment, and especially in cartilage regions with small focal defects. These data suggest that changes of T1 ρ values under mechanical loading may be related to the biomechanical and structural properties of cartilage. Hovis and colleagues[84] reported that light exercise was associated with low cartilage T2 values but moderate and strenuous exercise was associated with high T2 values in women, suggesting that activity levels can affect cartilage composition. In an interventional study assessing the effect of weight loss on articular cartilage, Anandacoomarasamy and colleagues[85] reported that improved articular cartilage quality was reflected as an increase in the dGEMRIC index over 1 year for the medial but not the lateral compartment. This finding highlights the role of weight loss in possible clinical and structural improvement.

Compositional changes in menisci may also be informative. Williams and colleagues[86] described intrameniscal biochemical alterations using ultrashort echo time-enhanced (UTE) T2* mapping, and found significant increases of UTE T2* values in the menisci of patients with anterior cruciate ligament injuries but with no clinical evidence of subsurface meniscal abnormality. UTE T2* is believed to reflect the integrity of the collagen network within the meniscus, and values are higher when there is collagen disorganization (ie, early meniscal damage).

Novel compositional techniques have been further explored. Raya and colleagues[87] found that in vivo diffusion tensor imaging based on a 7-T MR system could distinguish OA knees from non-OA knees better than T2 mapping. Other work on 7-T systems reported on the reproducibility of the method in vivo.[88] Other compositional techniques that might reward further exploration are T2* mapping[89] and sodium imaging[90] of cartilage. These techniques show promise, but they need to be practical and use standard MR imaging systems before they can be widely used for research or clinical diagnosis.

ULTRASONOGRAPHY

Ultrasonographic imaging enables real-time, multiplanar imaging at low cost. It offers reliable assessment of OA-associated features, including inflammatory and structural abnormalities, without contrast administration or exposure to radiation.[91] Limitations of ultrasonography include that it is an operator-dependent technique and that the physical properties of sound limit its ability to assess deep articular structures and the subchondral bone (**Fig. 12**).

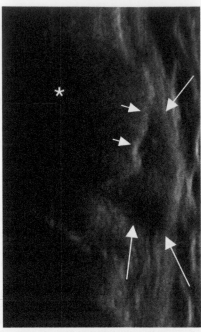

Fig. 12. Sonographic screenshot of the medial tibiofemoral joint space in advanced OA. Image depicts marked extrusion of the body of the medial meniscus (*long arrows*). Note that there is sound extinction at the osseous cortex (*small arrows*). As a consequence, the subchondral bone cannot be visualized (*asterisk*). Also the more central parts of the joint cavity itself including articular surfaces cannot be assessed.

Ultrasonography is useful for evaluation of cortical erosive changes and synovitis in inflammatory arthritis. In OA, the major advantage of ultrasonography over conventional radiography is the ability to detect synovial disease. Current-generation ultrasonographic technology can detect synovial hypertrophy, increased vascularity, and the presence of synovial fluid in joints affected by OA.[91] The Outcome Measures in Rheumatoid Arthritis Clinical Trials (OMERACT) Ultrasonography Taskforce defined synovial hypertrophy on ultrasonography as "abnormal hypoechoic (relative to subdermal fat, but sometimes may be isoechoic or hyperechoic) intra-articular tissue that is non-displaceable and poorly compressible and which may exhibit Doppler signal."[92] Although this definition was developed for use in rheumatoid arthritis, it may also be applied to OA, because the difference in synovial inflammation between OA and rheumatoid arthritis is largely quantitative rather than qualitative.[91]

The use of ultrasonography for imaging assessment of articular cartilage has been documented. Chiang and colleagues[93] reported a technique in which ultrasonography is used to detect surface fibrillatory changes (an early manifestation of OA) to accuracies of approximately 20 μm by taking advantage of the quantitative relationship between the surface roughness and angle-dependent acoustic backscatter. More recently, ultrasonographic elastography is used to study the depth-dependent elastic properties of cartilage structures to aid design and monitoring of engineered articular cartilage.[94] However, the use of these techniques in the context of OA imaging is still limited to the research environment.[95]

A preliminary ultrasonographic scoring system for features of hand OA published in 2008[96] included evaluation of gray-scale synovitis and power Doppler signal in

15 joints of the hand. These features were assessed for their presence/absence and, if present, were scored semiquantitatively using a 1 to 3 scale. Overall, the reliability exercise showed moderately good intrareader and interreader reliability. This study showed that an ultrasonographic outcome measure suitable for multicenter trials assessing hand OA is feasible and likely to be reliable and has provided a foundation for further development.

Ultrasonography has been increasingly used for assessment of hand OA. Kortekaas and colleagues[97] showed that ultrasound-detected osteophytes and JSN are associated with hand pain. The same group of investigators[98] also showed that signs of inflammation appear more frequently on ultrasonography in erosive OA hands than in nonerosive OA hands. This finding suggests the presence of an underlying systemic cause for erosive evolution. Klauser and colleagues[99] evaluated the efficacy of weekly ultrasound-guided intra-articular injections of hyaluronic acid. A decrease in pain correlated with a decrease in synovial thickening and power Doppler ultrasonography score before and after therapy. Iagnocco and colleagues[57] performed real-time fusion of ultrasonography and MR imaging in hand and wrist OA and found a high concordance of the bony profile visualization at the level of osteophytes.

Ultrasonography has also been used to evaluate features of knee OA[100,101] and hip OA.[102] A cross-sectional, multicenter European study supported by the European League Against Rheumatism analyzed 600 patients with painful knee OA and found that ultrasound-detected synovitis correlated with advanced radiographic OA and clinical symptoms and signs suggestive of an inflammatory flare.[100] Saarakkala and colleagues[101] evaluated the diagnostic performance of knee ultrasonography for the detection of degenerative changes of articular cartilage, using arthroscopic findings as the reference. These investigators found that positive ultrasonographic findings are strong indicators of cartilage degeneration, but negative findings do not exclude cartilage degeneration.

Wu and colleagues[103] investigated the association of ultrasonographic features with pain and functional scores in patients with equal radiographic grades of knee OA in both knees. These investigators showed that ultrasound-detected inflammatory features were positively and linearly associated with knee pain in motion. These findings confirmed the association between synovitis and knee pain, which has also been reported in MR imaging-based studies.[43] Ultrasonography has also been used to assess the clinical response to steroid injection,[104] but further studies are needed to show the usefulness of ultrasonography for this purpose.

NUCLEAR MEDICINE

In general, radioisotope methods provide imaging of active metabolism and enable visualization of bone turnover changes seen with osteophyte formation, subchondral sclerosis, subchondral cyst formation, and bone marrow lesions (all of which may be secondary to articular cartilage damage) as well as sites of synovitis.[105] Scintigraphy with technetium 99m-hydroxymethane diphosphonate and positron emission tomography (PET) with 2-^{18}F-fluoro-2-deoxy-D-glucose (18-FDG) or ^{18}F-fluoride (18-F$^-$) have been used to assess OA.[106] Bone scintigraphy is a simple examination that can provide a full-body survey that helps to discriminate between soft tissues and bone origin of pain, and to locate the site of pain in patients with complex symptoms.[106] 18-FDG PET can show the site of synovitis and bone marrow lesions associated with OA[107] and can also be used for bone imaging; the amount of tracer uptake depends on regional blood flow and bone remodeling conditions (**Fig. 13**).[108] An

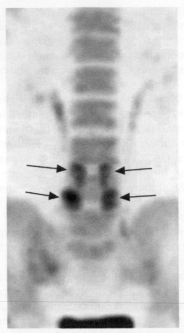

Fig. 13. Nuclear medicine. Coronal view of 18-FDG-PET examination shows marked glucose accumulation at the facet joints at L4 to L5 and L5 to S1 (*arrows*). This finding reflects hypermetabolism caused by circumscribed synovitis in facet joint OA.

in vivo study by Temmerman and colleagues[109] showed a significant increase in bone metabolism in the proximal femur of patients with symptomatic hip OA, showing that 18-F⁻ PET is a potentially useful technique for early detection of OA changes. Researchers are searching for a cartilage-specific radiopharmaceutical agent to be used with single-photon emission tomography for OA imaging.[110]

Limitations of radioisotope methods include poor anatomic resolution and the use of ionizing radiation. However, there are ways to overcome these issues. Hybrid technologies such as PET computed tomography (CT) and PET-MR imaging combine functional imaging with high-resolution anatomic imaging. A study by Moon and colleagues[111] showed that PET-CT could detect active inflammation in patients with OA of the shoulder. Techniques to achieve the optimum registration of PET and MR images are under development.[112] Although originally developed for breast imaging, small-part scanners may be useful for imaging of joints.[106] Small-part PET scanners have the advantages of lower operating costs and lower radiation exposure and retaining high spatial resolution and sensitivity for detection of lesions.

CT

CT is the method of choice for depicting cortical bone and soft tissue calcifications and has an established role in assessing facet joint OA of the spine in both clinical and research settings. Using a CT-based semiquantitative grading system of facet joint OA, Kalichman and colleagues[113] showed a high prevalence of facet joint OA, which increases with age and is most common at the L4 to L5 spinal level. In the same cohort, several associations were observed: self-reported back pain with spinal stenosis[114]; obesity with higher prevalence of facet joint OA[115]; and increasing age with higher prevalence of disk narrowing, facet joint OA, and degenerative spondylolisthesis (**Fig. 14**).[115] Kim and colleagues[116] used micro-CT to assess cartilage alterations in the facet joint of rats and showed that injection of monosodium iodoacetate into facet joints provided a useful model for the study of OA changes in the facet joint; they also showed that facet joint degeneration is a major cause of low back pain.

CT AND MR ARTHROGRAPHY

CT or MR arthrography enables evaluation of damage to articular cartilage with a high anatomic resolution in multiplanar fashion. CT arthrography can be performed using a single-contrast (iodine alone) or double-contrast (iodine and air) technique.[106] To avoid beam-hardening artifacts, the contrast material can be diluted with saline or local anesthetics.[106] For MR arthrography, gadolinium- diethylenetriamine pentaacetate (DTPA) is injected intra-articularly to visualize superficial cartilage defects. These arthrographic examinations have a low risk of infection from the intra-articular injection. Other risks include pain and vasovagal reactions, and systemic allergic reactions. CT arthrography exposes patients to radiation, but MR arthrography does not (**Fig. 15**).

CT arthrography is the most accurate method for evaluating articular cartilage surface damage. It offers high spatial resolution and high contrast between the

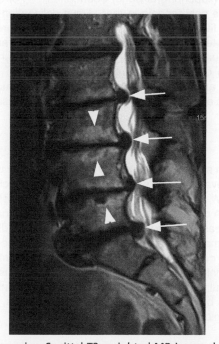

Fig. 14. OA of the lumbar spine. Sagittal T2-weighted MR image shows marked degenerative changes, including narrowing of the intervertebral spaces, disk bulging, and osseous end-plate changes representing lipomatous marrow conversion (Modic II changes [*arrowheads*]). Multisegmental spinal canal stenosis is observed as a result of disk alterations. Compared with CT, MR imaging better depicts soft tissue changes and bone marrow alterations.

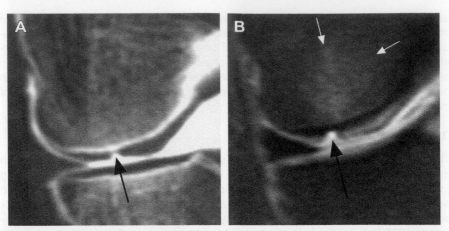

Fig. 15. Correlation of CT arthrography and MR imaging. (*A*) Coronal reformatted CT arthrography of the medial compartment shows a focal cartilage defect in the central femoral condyle (*arrow*). (*B*) Coronal fat-saturated T2-weighted MR image shows the same defect (*arrow*). In addition, the MR image depicts ill-defined subchondral bone marrow lesion not visualized on CT. (*Courtesy of* Prof Bruno Vande Berg, Brussels, Belgium.)

low-attenuating cartilage and high-attenuating superficial (contrast material filling the joint space) and deep (subchondral bone) boundaries.[106] For subchondral changes, MR arthrography is the only technique that allows delineation of subchondral bone marrow lesions on the fluid-sensitive sequences with fat suppression.[106] CT arthrography is ideally suited to depict subchondral bone sclerosis and osteophytes. Both techniques enable visualization of central osteophytes, which are associated with more severe changes of OA than marginal osteophytes.[117] Because of the high cost, invasive nature, and potential risk (albeit low) associated with intra-articular injection, arthrographic examinations are rarely used in large-scale clinical or epidemiologic OA studies.

SUMMARY

In clinical and research settings, radiography is still commonly used for semiquantitative and quantitative evaluation of structural OA features, such as osteophytes and JSN. Radiographic JSW measurement is still a recommended option for trials of structural modification in OA clinical trials, with the understanding that the concept of JSW represents several diseases, including cartilage and meniscal damage, and trial duration may be long. MR imaging is the most important imaging modality for research into OA, and investigators can select from semiquantitative, quantitative, and compositional assessment techniques. Ultrasonography is commonly used in hand OA studies and is particularly useful for evaluation of synovitis. Nuclear medicine, CT, and CT-MR arthrography can also be used for evaluation of OA features, but they have limited roles in large-scale clinical or epidemiologic studies.

REFERENCES

1. Altman RD, Gold GE. Atlas of individual radiographic features in osteoarthritis, revised. Osteoarthritis Cartilage 2007;15(Suppl A):A1–56.
2. Hunter DJ, Zhang YQ, Tu X, et al. Change in joint space width: hyaline articular cartilage loss or alteration in meniscus? Arthritis Rheum 2006;54:2488–95.

3. Altman R, Asch E, Bloch D, et al. Development of criteria for the classification and reporting of osteoarthritis. Classification of osteoarthritis of the knee. Diagnostic and Therapeutic Criteria Committee of the American Rheumatism Association. Arthritis Rheum 1986;29:1039–49.

4. Kinds MB, Vincken KL, Hoppinga TN, et al. Influence of variation in semiflexed knee positioning during image acquisition on separate quantitative radiographic parameters of osteoarthritis, measured by Knee Images Digital Analysis. Osteoarthritis Cartilage 2012;20:997–1003.

5. Kellgren JH, Lawrence JS. Radiological assessment of osteo-arthrosis. Ann Rheum Dis 1957;16:494–502.

6. Felson DT, Niu J, Guermazi A, et al. Defining radiographic incidence and progression of knee osteoarthritis: suggested modifications of the Kellgren and Lawrence scale. Ann Rheum Dis 2011;70:1884–6.

7. Felson DT, Nevitt MC, Yang M, et al. A new approach yields high rates of radiographic progression in knee osteoarthritis. J Rheumatol 2008;35:2047–54.

8. Guermazi A, Hunter DJ, Li L, et al. Different thresholds for detecting osteophytes and joint space narrowing exist between the site investigators and the centralized reader in a multicenter knee osteoarthritis study–data from the Osteoarthritis Initiative. Skeletal Radiol 2012;41:179–86.

9. Duryea J, Zaim S, Genant HK. New radiographic-based surrogate outcome measures for osteoarthritis of the knee. Osteoarthritis Cartilage 2003;11:102–10.

10. Chu E, DiCarlo JC, Peterfy C, et al. Fixed-location joint space width measurement increases sensitivity to change in osteoarthritis. Osteoarthritis Cartilage 2007;15:S192.

11. Nevitt MC, Peterfy C, Guermazi A, et al. Longitudinal performance evaluation and validation of fixed-flexion radiography of the knee for detection of joint space loss. Arthritis Rheum 2007;56:1512–20.

12. Duryea J, Neumann G, Niu J, et al. Comparison of radiographic joint space width with magnetic resonance imaging cartilage morphometry: analysis of longitudinal data from the Osteoarthritis Initiative. Arthritis Care Res (Hoboken) 2010;62:932–7.

13. Reichmann WM, Maillefert JF, Hunter DJ, et al. Responsiveness to change and reliability of measurement of radiographic joint space width in osteoarthritis of the knee: a systematic review. Osteoarthritis Cartilage 2011;19:550–6.

14. Mazzuca SA, Brandt KD, Chakr R, et al. Varus malalignment negates the structure-modifying benefits of doxycycline in obese women with knee osteoarthritis. Osteoarthritis Cartilage 2010;18:1008–11.

15. Kinds MB, Marijnissen AC, Vincken KL, et al. Evaluation of separate quantitative radiographic features adds to the prediction of incident radiographic osteoarthritis in individuals with recent onset of knee pain: 5-year follow-up in the CHECK cohort. Osteoarthritis Cartilage 2012;20:548–56.

16. Felson DT, Niu J, Gross KD, et al. Valgus malalignment is a risk factor for lateral knee osteoarthritis incidence and progression: findings from MOST and the Osteoarthritis Initiative. Arthritis Rheum 2013;65(2):355–62. http://dx.doi.org/10.1002/art.37726.

17. Woloszynski T, Podsiadlo P, Stachowiak GW, et al. Prediction of progression of radiographic knee osteoarthritis using tibial trabecular bone texture. Arthritis Rheum 2012;64:688–95.

18. Hayashi D, Xu L, Roemer FW, et al. Detection of osteophytes and subchondral cysts in the knee with use of tomosynthesis. Radiology 2012;263:206–15.

19. Conaghan PG, Hunter DJ, Maillefert JF, et al. Summary and recommendations of the OARSI FDA osteoarthritis Assessment of Structural Change Working Group. Osteoarthritis Cartilage 2011;19:606–10.
20. Eckstein F, Wirth W, Nevitt MC. Recent advances in osteoarthritis imaging–the Osteoarthritis Initiative. Nat Rev Rheumatol 2012;8:622–30.
21. Hayashi D, Guermazi A, Roemer FW. MRI of osteoarthritis: the challenges of definition and quantification. Semin Musculoskelet Radiol 2012;16:419–30.
22. Guermazi A, Niu J, Hayashi D, et al. Prevalence of abnormalities in knees detected by MRI in adults without knee osteoarthritis: population based observational study (Framingham Osteoarthritis Study). BMJ 2012;345:e5339.
23. Englund M, Roemer FW, Hayashi D, et al. Meniscus pathology, osteoarthritis and the treatment controversy. Nat Rev Rheumatol 2012;8:412–9.
24. Hayashi D, Roemer FW, Dhina Z, et al. Longitudinal assessment of cyst-like lesions of the knee and their relation to radiographic osteoarthritis and MRI-detected effusion and synovitis in patients with knee pain. Arthritis Res Ther 2010;12:R172.
25. Hayashi D, Guermazi A, Kwoh CK, et al. Semiquantitative assessment of subchondral bone marrow edema-like lesions and subchondral cysts of the knee at 3T MRI: a comparison between intermediate-weighted fat-suppressed spin echo and Dual Echo Steady State sequences. BMC Musculoskelet Disord 2011;12:198.
26. Hayashi D, Englund M, Roemer FW, et al. Knee malalignment is associated with an increased risk for incident and enlarging bone marrow lesions in the more loaded compartments: the MOST study. Osteoarthritis Cartilage 2012;20:1227–33.
27. Roemer FW, Felson DT, Wang K, et al. Co-localisation of non-cartilaginous articular pathology increases risk of cartilage loss in the tibiofemoral joint–the MOST study. Ann Rheum Dis 2012. [Epub ahead of print].
28. Crema MD, Roemer FW, Felson DT, et al. Factors associated with meniscal extrusion in knees with or at risk for osteoarthritis: the Multicenter Osteoarthritis study. Radiology 2012;264:494–503.
29. Roemer FW, Guermazi A, Felson DT, et al. Risk factors for magnetic resonance imaging-detected patellofemoral and tibiofemoral cartilage loss during a six-month period: the joints on glucosamine study. Arthritis Rheum 2012;64:1888–98.
30. Roemer FW, Guermazi A, Felson DT, et al. Presence of MRI-detected joint effusion and synovitis increases the risk of cartilage loss in knees without osteoarthritis at 30-month follow-up: the MOST study. Ann Rheum Dis 2011;70:1804–9.
31. Englund M, Felson DT, Guermazi A, et al. Risk factors for medial meniscal pathology on knee MRI in older US adults: a multicentre prospective cohort study. Ann Rheum Dis 2011;70:1733–9.
32. Felson DT, Parkes MJ, Marjanovic EJ, et al. Bone marrow lesions in knee osteoarthritis change in 6–12 weeks. Osteoarthritis Cartilage 2012;20:1514–8.
33. Crema MD, Felson DT, Roemer FW, et al. Prevalent cartilage damage and cartilage loss over time are associated with incident bone marrow lesions in the tibiofemoral compartments: the MOST study. Osteoarthritis Cartilage 2013;21(2):306–13. http://dx.doi.org/10.1016/j.joca.2012.11.005.
34. Hunter DJ. Insights from imaging on the epidemiology and pathophysiology of osteoarthritis. Radiol Clin North Am 2009;47:539–51.
35. von Engelhardt LV, Kraft CN, Pennekamp PH, et al. The evaluation of articular cartilage lesions of the knee with a 3-Tesla magnet. Arthroscopy 2007;23:496–502.

36. Madhusudhan TR, Kumar TM, Bastawrous SS, et al. Clinical examination, MRI and arthroscopy in meniscal and ligamentous knee injuries–a prospective study. J Orthop Surg Res 2008;3:19.
37. Quatman CE, Hettrich CM, Schmitt LC, et al. The clinical utility and diagnostic performance of magnetic resonance imaging for identification of early and advanced knee osteoarthritis: a systematic review. Am J Sports Med 2011;39: 1557–68.
38. Hayashi D, Jarraya M, Guermazi A, et al. Frequency and fluctuation of susceptibility artifacts in the tibiofemoral joint space in painful knees on 3T MRI and association with meniscal tears, radiographic joint space narrowing and calcifications. Arthritis Rheum 2012;64(Suppl 10):1030.
39. Hunter DJ, Arden N, Conaghan P, et al. Definition of osteoarthritis on MRI: results of a Delphi exercise. Osteoarthritis Cartilage 2011;19:963–9.
40. Roemer FW, Guermazi A, Niu J, et al. Prevalence of magnetic resonance imaging-defined atrophic and hypertrophic phenotypes of knee osteoarthritis in a population-based cohort. Arthritis Rheum 2012;64:429–37.
41. Zhang Y, Nevitt M, Niu J, et al. Fluctuation of knee pain and changes in bone marrow lesions, effusions, and synovitis on magnetic resonance imaging. Arthritis Rheum 2011;63:691–9.
42. Felson DT, Chaisson CE, Hill CL, et al. The association of bone marrow lesions with pain in knee osteoarthritis. Ann Intern Med 2001;134:541–9.
43. Guermazi A, Roemer FW, Hayashi D, et al. Assessment of synovitis with contrast-enhanced MRI using a whole-joint semiquantitative scoring system in people with, or at high risk of, knee osteoarthritis: the MOST study. Ann Rheum Dis 2011;70:805–11.
44. Hunter DJ, Zhang W, Conaghan PG, et al. Systematic review of the concurrent and predictive validity of MRI biomarkers in OA. Osteoarthritis Cartilage 2011; 19:557–88.
45. Hunter DJ, Zhang W, Conaghan PG, et al. Responsiveness and reliability of MRI in knee osteoarthritis: a meta-analysis of published evidence. Osteoarthritis Cartilage 2011;19:589–605.
46. Guermazi A, Roemer FW, Haugen IK, et al. MRI-based semiquantitative scoring of joint pathology in osteoarthritis. Nat Rev Rheumatol 2013. http://dx.doi.org/10.1038/nrrheum.2012.223.
47. Peterfy CG, Guermazi A, Zaim S, et al. Whole-Organ Magnetic Resonance Imaging Score (WORMS) of the knee in osteoarthritis. Osteoarthritis Cartilage 2004;12:177–90.
48. Kornaat PR, Ceulemans RY, Kroon HM, et al. MRI assessment of knee osteoarthritis: Knee Osteoarthritis Scoring System (KOSS)–inter-observer and intraobserver reproducibility of a compartment-based scoring system. Skeletal Radiol 2005;34:95–102.
49. Hunter DJ, Lo GH, Gale D, et al. The reliability of a new scoring system for knee osteoarthritis MRI and the validity of bone marrow lesion assessment: BLOKS (Boston Leeds Osteoarthritis Knee Score). Ann Rheum Dis 2008;67:206–11.
50. Hunter DJ, Guermazi A, Lo GH, et al. Evolution of semi-quantitative whole joint assessment of knee OA: MOAKS (MRI Osteoarthritis Knee Score). Osteoarthritis Cartilage 2011;19:990–1002.
51. Lynch JA, Roemer FW, Nevitt MC, et al. Comparison of BLOKS and WORMS scoring systems part I. Cross sectional comparison of methods to assess cartilage morphology, meniscal damage and bone marrow lesions on knee MRI: data from the osteoarthritis initiative. Osteoarthritis Cartilage 2010;18:1393–401.

52. Felson DT, Lynch J, Guermazi A, et al. Comparison of BLOKS and WORMS scoring systems part II. Longitudinal assessment of knee MRIs for osteoarthritis and suggested approach based on their performance: data from the Osteoarthritis Initiative. Osteoarthritis Cartilage 2010;18:1402–7.

53. Roemer FW, Nevitt MC, Felson DT, et al. Predictive validity of within-grade scoring of longitudinal changes of MRI-based cartilage morphology and bone marrow lesion assessment in the tibio-femoral joint–the MOST Study. Osteoarthritis Cartilage 2012;20(11):1391–8.

54. Bloecker K, Guermazi A, Wirth W, et al. Tibial coverage, meniscus position, size and damage in knees discordant for joint space narrowing–data from the Osteoarthritis Initiative. Osteoarthritis Cartilage 2013;21(3):419–27.

55. Baker K, Grainger A, Niu J, et al. Relation of synovitis to knee pain using contrast-enhanced MRIs. Ann Rheum Dis 2010;69:1779–83.

56. Loeuille D, Sauliere N, Champigneulle J, et al. Comparing non-enhanced and enhanced sequences in the assessment of effusion and synovitis in knee OA: associations with clinical, macroscopic and microscopic features. Osteoarthritis Cartilage 2011;19:1433–9.

57. Iagnocco A, Perella C, D'Agostino MA, et al. Magnetic resonance and ultrasonography real-time fusion imaging of the hand and wrist in osteoarthritis and rheumatoid arthritis. Rheumatology (Oxford) 2011;50:1409–13.

58. Wittoek R, Jans L, Lambrecht V, et al. Reliability and construct validity of ultrasonography of soft tissue and destructive changes in erosive osteoarthritis of the interphalangeal finger joints: a comparison with MRI. Ann Rheum Dis 2011;70:278–83.

59. Haugen IK, Lillegraven S, Slatkowsky-Christensen B, et al. Hand osteoarthritis and MRI: development and first validation step of the proposed Oslo Hand Osteoarthritis MRI score. Ann Rheum Dis 2011;70:1033–8.

60. Haugen IK, Boyesen P, Slatkowsky-Christensen B, et al. Comparison of features by MRI and radiographs of the interphalangeal finger joints in patients with hand osteoarthritis. Ann Rheum Dis 2012;71:345–50.

61. Haugen IK, Boyesen P, Slatkowsky-Christensen B, et al. Associations between MRI-defined synovitis, bone marrow lesions and structural features and measures of pain and physical function in hand osteoarthritis. Ann Rheum Dis 2012;71:899–904.

62. Roemer FW, Hunter DJ, Winterstein A, et al. Hip Osteoarthritis MRI Scoring System (HOAMS): reliability and associations with radiographic and clinical findings. Osteoarthritis Cartilage 2011;19:946–62.

63. Eckstein F, Ateshian G, Burgkart R, et al. Proposal for a nomenclature for magnetic resonance imaging based measures of articular cartilage in osteoarthritis. Osteoarthritis Cartilage 2006;14:974–83.

64. Buck RJ, Wyman BT, Le Graverand MP, et al. An efficient subset of morphological measures for articular cartilage in the healthy and diseased human knee. Magn Reson Med 2010;63:680–90.

65. Buck RJ, Wyman BT, Le Graverand MP, et al. Does the use of ordered values of subregional change in cartilage thickness improve the detection of disease progression in longitudinal studies of osteoarthritis? Arthritis Rheum 2009;61: 917–24.

66. Wirth W, Buck R, Nevitt M, et al. MRI-based extended ordered values more efficiently differentiate cartilage loss in knees with and without joint space narrowing than region-specific approaches using MRI or radiography–data from the OA initiative. Osteoarthritis Cartilage 2011;19:689–99.

67. Bennell KL, Bowles KA, Wang Y, et al. Higher dynamic medial knee load predicts greater cartilage loss over 12 months in medial knee osteoarthritis. Ann Rheum Dis 2011;70:1770–4.
68. Eckstein F, Cotofana S, Wirth W, et al. Greater rates of cartilage loss in painful knees than in pain-free knees after adjustment for radiographic disease stage: data from the osteoarthritis initiative. Arthritis Rheum 2011;63:2257–67.
69. Eckstein F, Nevitt M, Gimona A, et al. Rates of change and sensitivity to change in cartilage morphology in healthy knees and in knees with mild, moderate, and end-stage radiographic osteoarthritis: results from 831 participants from the Osteoarthritis Initiative. Arthritis Care Res (Hoboken) 2011;63: 311–9.
70. Eckstein F, Kwoh CK, Boudreau RM, et al. Quantitative MRI measures of cartilage predict knee replacement: a case-control study from the Osteoarthritis Initiative. Ann Rheum Dis 2012. [Epub ahead of print].
71. Schneider E, Nevitt M, McCulloch C, et al. Equivalence and precision of knee cartilage morphometry between different segmentation teams, cartilage regions, and MR acquisitions. Osteoarthritis Cartilage 2012;20:869–79.
72. Wirth W, Frobell RB, Souza RB, et al. A three-dimensional quantitative method to measure meniscus shape, position, and signal intensity using MR images: a pilot study and preliminary results in knee osteoarthritis. Magn Reson Med 2010;63: 1162–71.
73. Siorpaes K, Wenger A, Bloecker K, et al. Interobserver reproducibility of quantitative meniscus analysis using coronal multiplanar DESS and IWTSE MR imaging. Magn Reson Med 2012;67:1419–26.
74. Wenger A, Englund M, Wirth W, et al. Relationship of 3D meniscal morphology and position with knee pain in subjects with knee osteoarthritis: a pilot study. Eur Radiol 2012;22:211–20.
75. Roemer FW, Khrad H, Hayashi D, et al. Volumetric and semiquantitative assessment of MRI-detected subchondral bone marrow lesions in knee osteoarthritis: a comparison of contrast-enhanced and non-enhanced imaging. Osteoarthritis Cartilage 2010;18:1062–6.
76. Fotinos-Hoyer AK, Guermazi A, Jara H, et al. Assessment of synovitis in the osteoarthritic knee: comparison between manual segmentation, semi-automated segmentation and semiquantitative assessment using contrast-enhanced fat-suppressed T1-weighted MRI. Magn Reson Med 2010;64:604–9.
77. Habib S, Guermazi A, Ozonoff A, et al. MRI-based volumetric assessment of joint effusion in knee osteoarthritis using proton density-weighted fat-suppressed and T1-weighted contrast-enhanced fat-suppressed sequences. Skeletal Radiol 2011;40:1581–5.
78. Burstein D, Gray M, Mosher T, et al. Measures of molecular composition and structure in osteoarthritis. Radiol Clin North Am 2009;47:675–86.
79. Crema MD, Roemer FW, Marra MD, et al. Articular cartilage in the knee: current MR imaging techniques and applications in clinical practice and research. Radiographics 2011;31:37–61.
80. Roos EM, Dahlberg L. Positive effects of moderate exercise on glycosaminoglycan content in knee cartilage: a four-month, randomized, controlled trial in patients at risk of osteoarthritis. Arthritis Rheum 2005;52:3507–14.
81. McAlindon TE, Nuite M, Krishnan N, et al. Change in knee osteoarthritis cartilage detected by delayed gadolinium enhanced magnetic resonance imaging following treatment with collagen hydrolysate: a pilot randomized controlled trial. Osteoarthritis Cartilage 2011;19:399–405.

82. Van Ginckel A, Baelde N, Almqvist KM, et al. Functional adaptation of knee carti-lage in asymptomatic female novice runners compared to sedentary controls. A longitudinal analysis using delayed Gadolinium Enhanced Magnetic Resonance Imaging of Cartilage (dGEMRIC). Osteoarthritis Cartilage 2010;18:1564–9.
83. Souza RB, Stehling C, Wyman BT, et al. The effects of acute loading on T1rho and T2 relaxation times of tibiofemoral articular cartilage. Osteoarthritis Carti-lage 2010;18:1557–63.
84. Hovis KK, Stehling C, Souza RB, et al. Physical activity is associated with magnetic resonance imaging-based knee cartilage T2 measurements in asymp-tomatic subjects with and those without osteoarthritis risk factors. Arthritis Rheum 2011;63:2248–56.
85. Anandacoomarasamy A, Leibman S, Smith G, et al. Weight loss in obese people has structure-modifying effects on medial but not on lateral knee articular carti-lage. Ann Rheum Dis 2012;71:26–32.
86. Wiliams A, Qian Y, Golla S, et al. UTE-T2* mapping detects sub-clinical meniscus injury after anterior cruciate ligament tear. Osteoarthritis Cartilage 2012;20:486–94.
87. Raya JG, Horng A, Dietrich O, et al. Articular cartilage: in vivo diffusion-tensor imaging. Radiology 2012;262:550–9.
88. Madelin G, Babb JS, Xia D, et al. Reproducibility and repeatability of quantita-tive sodium magnetic resonance imaging in vivo in articular cartilage at 3 T and 7 T. Magn Reson Med 2012;68:841–9.
89. Newbould RD, Miller SR, Toms LD, et al. T2* measurement of the knee articular cartilage in osteoarthritis at 3T. J Magn Reson Imaging 2012;35:1422–9.
90. Lesperance LM, Gray ML, Burstein D. Determination of fixed charge density in cartilage using nuclear magnetic resonance. J Orthop Res 1922;10:1–13.
91. Keen HI, Conaghan PG. Ultrasonography in osteoarthritis. Radiol Clin North Am 2009;47:581–94.
92. Wakefield RJ, Balint P, Szkudlarek M, et al. Musculoskeletal ultrasound including definitions for ultrasonographic pathology. J Rheumatol 2005;32:2485–7.
93. Chiang EH, Laing TJ, Meyer CR, et al. Ultrasonic characterization of in vitro oste-oarthritis articular cartilage with validation by confocal microscopy. Ultrasound Med Biol 1997;23:205–13.
94. McCredie AJ, Stride E, Saffari N. Ultrasound elastography to determine the layered mechanical properties of articular cartilage and the importance of such structural characteristics under load. Conf Proc IEEE Eng Med Biol Soc 2009; 2009:4262–5.
95. Drakonaki EE, Allen GM, Wilson DJ. Ultrasound elastography for musculoskel-etal applications. Br J Radiol 2012;85:1435–45.
96. Keen HI, Lavie F, Wakefield RJ, et al. The development of a preliminary ultraso-nographic scoring system for features of hand osteoarthritis. Ann Rheum Dis 2008;67:651–5.
97. Kortekaas MC, Kwok WY, Reijnierse M, et al. Osteophytes and joint space nar-rowing are independently associated with pain in finger joints in hand osteoar-thritis. Ann Rheum Dis 2011;70:1835–7.
98. Kortekaas MC, Kwok WY, Reijnierse M, et al. In erosive hand osteoarthritis more inflammatory signs on ultrasound are found than in the rest of hand osteoar-thritis. Ann Rheum Dis 2012. [Epub ahead of print].
99. Klauser AS, Faschingbauer R, Kupferthaler K, et al. Sonographic criteria for therapy follow-up in the course of ultrasound-guided intra-articular injections of hyaluronic acid in hand osteoarthritis. Eur J Radiol 2012;81:1607–11.

100. Conaghan PG, D'Agostino MA, Le Bars M, et al. Clinical and ultrasonographic predictors of joint replacement for knee osteoarthritis: results from a large, 3-year, prospective EULAR study. Ann Rheum Dis 2010;69:644–7.

101. Saarakkala S, Waris P, Waris V, et al. Diagnostic performance of knee ultrasonography for detecting degenerative changes of articular cartilage. Osteoarthritis Cartilage 2012;20:376–81.

102. Iagnocco A, Filippucci E, Riente L, et al. Ultrasound imaging for the rheumatologist XLI. Sonographic assessment of the hip in OA patients. Clin Exp Rheumatol 2012;30:652–7.

103. Wu PT, Shao CJ, Wu KC, et al. Pain in patients with equal radiographic grades of osteoarthritis in both knees: the value of gray scale ultrasound. Osteoarthritis Cartilage 2012;20:1507–13.

104. Chao J, Wu C, Sun B, et al. Inflammatory characteristics on ultrasound predict poorer longterm response to intraarticular corticosteroid injections in knee osteoarthritis. J Rheumatol 2010;37:650–5.

105. Etchebehere EC, Etchebehere M, Gamba R, et al. Orthopedic pathology of the lower extremities: scintigraphic evaluation in the thigh, knee and leg. Semin Nucl Med 1998;28:41–61.

106. Omoumi P, Mercier GA, Lecouvet F, et al. CT arthrography, MR arthrography, PET and scintigraphy in osteoarthritis. Radiol Clin North Am 2009;47:595–615.

107. Nakamura H, Masuko K, Yudoh K, et al. Positron emission tomography with 18F-FDG in osteoarthritic knee. Osteoarthritis Cartilage 2007;15:673–81.

108. Umemoto Y, Oka T, Inoue T, et al. Imaging of a rat osteoarthritis model using (18) F-fluoride positron emission tomography. Ann Nucl Med 2010;24:663–9.

109. Temmerman OP, Raijmakers PG, Kloet R, et al. In vivo measurements of blood flow and bone metabolism in osteoarthritis. Rheumatol Int 2012. [Epub ahead of print].

110. Cachin F, Boisgard S, Vidal A, et al. First ex vivo study demonstrating that 99mTc-NTP 15–5 radiotracer binds to human articular cartilage. Eur J Nucl Med Mol Imaging 2011;38:2077–82.

111. Moon YL, Lee SH, Park SY, et al. Evaluation of shoulder disorders by 2-[F-18]-fluoro-2-deoxy-D-glucose positron emission tomography and computed tomography. Clin Orthop Surg 2010;2:167–72.

112. Magee D, Tanner SF, Waller M, et al. Combining variational and model-based techniques to register PET and MR images in hand osteoarthritis. Phys Med Biol 2010;55:4755–69.

113. Kalichman L, Li L, Kim DH, et al. Facet joint osteoarthritis and low back pain in the community-based population. Spine 2008;33:2560–5.

114. Kalichman L, Kim DH, Li L, et al. Computed tomography evaluated features of spinal degeneration: prevalence, intercorrelation, and association with self-reported low back pain. Spine 2010;10:200–8.

115. Kalichman L, Guermazi A, Li L, et al. Association between age, sex, BMI and CT-evaluated spinal degeneration features. J Back Musculoskelet Rehabil 2009;22:189–95.

116. Kim JS, Kroin JS, Buvanendran A, et al. Characterization of a new animal model for evaluation and treatment of back pain due to lumbar facet joint osteoarthritis. Arthritis Rheum 2011;63:2966–73.

117. McCauley TR, Kornaat PR, Jee WH. Central osteophytes in the knee: prevalence and association with cartilage defects on MR imaging. AJR Am J Roentgenol 2001;176:359–64.

Role of Imaging in the Diagnosis of Large and Medium-Sized Vessel Vasculitis

Nicolò Pipitone, MD, PhD[a], Annibale Versari, MD[b],
Gene G. Hunder, MD[c], Carlo Salvarani, MD[a],*

KEYWORDS

- Vasculitis • Tomography radiograph computed • Magnetic resonance imaging
- Ultrasonography • Positron emission tomography

KEY POINTS

- In large-vessel vasculitis, imaging studies are useful to document temporal artery involvement and crucial to demonstrate large-vessel involvement.
- Color Doppler sonography, magnetic resonance, and computed tomography are able to show early vasculitic lesions, characterized by inflammatory vessel wall alterations with initial sparing of the vessel lumen.
- In contrast, angiography delineates well later vascular complications such as stenoses, occlusions, and aneurysms, but cannot show early vasculitic lesions such as vessel wall alterations.
- Positron emission tomography is very sensitive in detecting large-vessel inflammation, but cannot delineate the anatomic details of the vessels involved.
- Imaging techniques are useful in the work-up of large-vessel and medium-vessel vasculitis.

INTRODUCTION

Primary systemic vasculitides (PSV) are usually classified by the diameter of the vessels that are predominantly involved, although additional refining parameters are the presence of granulomata and the positivity of antineutrophil cytoplasmic antibodies (ANCA).[1] Large-vessel vasculitides (LVV) include giant cell arteritis (GCA),

[a] Rheumatology Unit, Department of Internal Medicine, Azienda Ospedaliera ASMN, Istituto di Ricovero e Cura a Carattere Scientifico, Viale Risorgimento 80, Reggio Emilia 42123, Italy; [b] Nuclear Medicine Unit, Department of Advanced Technology, Azienda Ospedaliera ASMN, Istituto di Ricovero e Cura a Carattere Scientifico, Reggio Emilia, Italy; [c] Division of Rheumatology, Department of Medicine, Mayo Clinic College of Medicine, 200 First Street South West, Rochester, MN 55905, USA
* Corresponding author. Department of Rheumatology, Arcispedale Santa Maria Nuova, Viale Risorgimento 80, Reggio Emilia 42123, Italy.
E-mail address: salvarani.carlo@asmn.re.it

Rheum Dis Clin N Am 39 (2013) 593–608
http://dx.doi.org/10.1016/j.rdc.2013.02.002
0889-857X/13/$ – see front matter © 2013 Elsevier Inc. All rights reserved.

Takayasu arteritis (TAK), primary central nervous system vasculitis (PCNSV), and chronic periaortitis (CP). Medium-vessel vasculitides are classically represented by polyarteritis nodosa (PAN) in adults and Kawasaki disease (KD) in children, whereas ANCA-associated vasculitides (AAV) can affect both medium and small vessels. Imaging techniques are particularly useful to diagnose and monitor LVV, but play also a key role in the work-up of medium-vessel vasculitides. In contrast, they are unable to visualize small vessels. This review focuses on the role of imaging studies in diagnosing and monitoring LVV, but also mention their principal applications in medium-vessel vasculitides.

LVV: GCA AND TAK

GCA and TAK are LVV mainly involving the aorta and its main branches. Compared with TAK, GCA has a predilection for the temporal arteries (TA) and other extracranial arteries and affects more often the axillary arteries, but overall the distribution of arteries affected largely overlaps.[2]

Early LVV is characterized by vessel wall inflammatory lesions (thickening and mural edema), with initial sparing of the arterial lumen. Color Doppler sonography (CDS), magnetic resonance (MR), and computed tomography (CT) are all able to depict the vessel wall and thus to secure an early diagnosis of LVV. Increased vessel wall thickness with a hypoechoic halo on CDS, or vessel wall edema and mural enhancement on CT or MR, are signs of active vasculitis.[3]

CDS

The use of CDS in GCA was spearheaded in 1997 by Schmidt and colleagues,[4] who showed that inflamed TA were characterized by a hypoechoic concentric wall thickening, dubbed halo sign (**Fig. 1**). The investigators reported a specificity of ~100% and a sensitivity of 73% of the halo sign for the diagnosis of GCA, whereas stenoses and occlusions, albeit common (80% of cases), were less sensitive and specific. Since then, CDS of the TA has increasingly been used to screen for suspected GCA. According to a recent meta-analysis, the presence of a halo in the TA has a sensitivity of 75% and a specificity of 83% for the diagnosis of GCA using the histologic criteria as

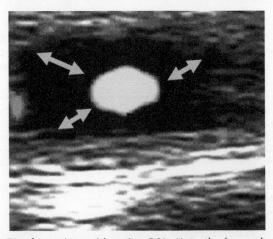

Fig. 1. CDS of the TA of a patient with active GCA. Note the hypoechoic halo (halo sign, *double arrows*) surrounding the arterial lumen.

reference standard,[5] and a sensitivity of 68% and specificity of 91% for GCA diagnosed according to the American College of Rheumatology (ACR) criteria.[6] The specificity of the halo sign increases to nearly 100% when the sign is bilateral.[6] However, findings of TA CDS do not predict ocular complications.[7]

The halo sign can also be noted in inflamed large vessels in GCA.[8] In 3 studies that investigated the occurrence of large-vessel inflammation in GCA, ~30% of unselected patients with new onset of GCA had CDS evidence of LVV (ie, a positive halo sign).[9–11] In clinical practice, CDS of the epiaortic (carotid, subclavian, and axillary) arteries probably suffices in most cases to establish whether a patient with GCA has LVV, because aortitis or lower-limb arteritis rarely occurs in the absence of epiaortic arteritis.[9,12]

The equivalent of the halo sign in TAK is the macaroni sign, a circumferential midechoic vessel wall thickening.[13] Compared with the halo sign, the macaroni sign is on average brighter, probably reflecting less acute inflammation.[14] As in large-vessel GCA, CDS is a valuable screening test for suspected TAK. In this regard, in one study,[15] CDS of the carotid arteries was able to detect a thickened vessel wall in 28 of 44 carotid arteries from 44 patients with TAK, whereas conventional angiography could depict stenoses in only 21 arteries.

Recently, the use of a contrast agent has been suggested to improve the quality of ultrasonographic images and to provide an additional measure of vascular inflammation before and after treatment.[16,17] However, it is unclear whether enhanced CDS provides a significant advantage over standard CDS in diagnosing and monitoring LVV.

Because CDS can depict not only the vessel wall but also the lumen, it lends itself well to monitoring vascular complications of LVV such as stenoses or aneurysms in accessible vessels.[3] Vessel wall thickening often persists even after successful therapy, whereas the halo sign usually resolves after variable periods of time (1–32 weeks).[4,18] The halo sign may resolve more quickly in the TA than in large vessels.[19] In a recent study using histology as reference, TA CDS performed 0 to 1 days after onset of glucocorticoid (GC) therapy showed 92% sensitivity and 57% specificity for GCA, whereas when CDS was performed over 4 days after onset of GC therapy, sensitivity and specificity dropped to 50% and 25%, respectively.[20]

Advantages of CDS include its higher (~10-fold) resolution compared with MR, its limited costs, the short time required for image acquisition, and the absence of exposure to ionizing radiation.[3,21] Limitations of CDS include the lack of visualization of the thoracic aorta, poor visualization of the abdominal aorta, and a substantial degree of operator dependency, although adequate training in vascular CDS has been shown to produce excellent interreader and intrareader agreement, with κ coefficients of 0.848 and 0.950, respectively.[22]

CT and CT Angiography

CT is well suited to detect inflammatory changes in large, deep arteries such as the aorta (**Fig. 2**).[3] In early LVV, CT typically shows thickening of the arterial wall with mural enhancement, whereas CT angiography (CTA) can detect late vascular complications.[23,24] Mural enhancement usually resolves or markedly improves after successful treatment, although its improvement may lag behind clinical and laboratory improvement.[25,26] Compared with conventional angiography, CTA has been shown to be able to accurately assess stenotic lesions in TAK in all brachiocephalic trunks, in 37 of 40 common carotid arteries, and in 33 of 40 subclavian arteries, with a sensitivity and specificity of 93% and 98%, respectively.[27] Likewise, in GCA, CTA was able to detect large-vessel involvement in 27 of 40 patients; the aorta (65% of patients), the brachiocephalic trunk (48%), the carotid arteries (35%), and the subclavian arteries (43%)

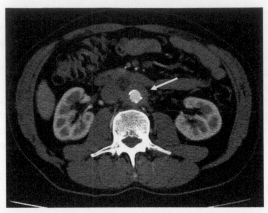

Fig. 2. CT scan showing circumferential thickening of the abdominal aorta (*arrow*) in a patient with large-vessel vasculitis. (*Courtesy of* Dr Lucia Spaggiari, MD, Radiology Department, Arcispedale Santa Maria Nuova, Reggio Emilia, Italy.)

were mainly affected.[28] The main disadvantage of CT/CTA is the exposure to a significant amount of ionizing radiation,[3] which limits its repeated use, especially in young individuals.

MR and MR Angiography

Similarly to CT, MR is particularly indicated to examine the aorta and other deep, large vessels (**Fig. 3**A). A sign of early vasculitis is increased thickness of the arterial wall, usually with a diffuse pattern, associated with edema of the vessel wall (in T2 and fat-suppressed sequences) or mural enhancement (in T1-weighted sequences).[29,30] Postcontrast T1 images are superior to T2 or fat-suppressed images to detect large-vessel inflammation. In this regard, a study that compared 3-T MR T2-weighted inversion recovery (IR) fast spin echo (SE) images with postcontrast

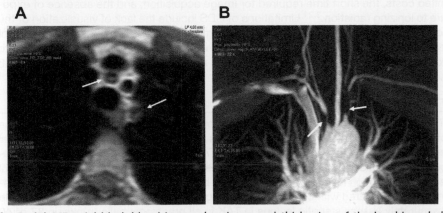

Fig. 3. (*A*) MR axial black blood image showing mural thickening of the brachiocephalic trunk and of the left subclavian artery (*arrows*) in a patient with TAK. (*B*) MR angiography of the same patient of Fig. 3A. On the right, note the stenosis of the brachiocephalic trunk, and on the left, the subclavian artery is occluded. (*Courtesy of* Dr Lucia Spaggiari, MD, Radiology Department, Arcispedale Santa Maria Nuova, Reggio Emilia, Italy.)

T1-weighted SE images showed that only marked inflammatory signs could be appreciated using T2 IR fast SE sequences, whereas detection of more subtle signs required the use of postcontrast images.[31]

MR has also been used to examine the TA in patients with GCA. We previously showed that enhanced, low-resolution 1-T MR of the TA had a high specificity (100%) but low sensitivity (28%) to show inflammation of the TA in GCA.[32] On the contrary, high-resolution 1.5-T MR of the TA has been shown to be 81% sensitive and 97% specific for GCA using the ACR classification criteria as reference standard.[33] The limited sensitivity of MR in this setting is probably largely caused by the lack of or only minor involvement of the TA in a subset of patients with GCA.[34]

MR is often combined with MR angiography (MRA) to visualize the vascular lumen (see **Fig. 3**B).[23] Similarly to CTA, MRA poorly visualizes smaller vessels, whereas stenoses may be falsely accentuated.[23,35] However, because small vessels are not affected by GCA or TAK, for practical purposes, the sensitivity of MRA in LVV is equal to that of conventional angiography.[36]

Like other imaging techniques, MR has only a limited predictive power for the development of vascular lesions. In a study of 24 patients with TAK, 6 of 16 patients had no disease progression despite persistent vessel wall edema, whereas 3 patients developed new lesions at sites without vessel wall edema.[37]

MR findings can be affected by GC therapy. In a study, high-resolution MR of the TA was performed in 17 patients with proven GCA at the onset of GC treatment and after 16 months of therapy. Intensity of inflammatory enhancement decreased significantly under GC therapy.[38] Similarly, sequential MR images of the cranial and epiaortic arteries obtained from patients with biopsy-proven GCA during GC therapy showed a decrease in mural inflammation within the first 2 weeks and an almost complete resolution after 2.5 months of continued treatment.[39] Improvement of vascular stenotic lesions after the institution of immunosuppressive treatment has also been shown using MRA.[39,40]

Digital Subtraction Angiography

Digital subtraction angiography (DSA) clearly shows alterations of the vessel lumen, but cannot show early vasculitic lesions such as thickening of the vessel wall, and is therefore not useful to make an early diagnosis of LVV.[3] In contrast, serial angiograms can be used to determine the evolution of vascular complications such as stenoses or aneurysms.[35] In addition, DSA still has a role in guiding interventional procedure like placement of stents. DSA involves exposure to ionizing radiation, required invasive cannulation via femoral access, and carries a small risk of complications, including permanent stroke (0.25%).[41]

18F-Fluorodeoxyglucose Positron Emission Tomography

Positron emission tomography (PET) is a nuclear medicine technique that is able to evaluate the degree of vascular uptake of a radiolabeled glucose analogue (fluorodeoxyglucose [FDG]) by activated cells in infections, malignancies, and inflammatory processes.[3] In large vessels, the intensity of FDG uptake is usually classified on a semiquantitative 4-point scale: none (grade 0), less than liver uptake (grade 1), similar to liver uptake (grade 2), and higher than liver uptake (grade 3).[42] Grades 2 to 3 are relatively specific for vasculitis.[43] Alternatively, an aorta-to-liver maximal standardized uptake value cutoff ratio of 1.0 has proved highly sensitive (89%) and specific (95%) for GCA-related large-vessel inflammation.[44] Overall, according to a recent meta-analysis, PET has a sensitivity of 80% and a specificity of 89% for the diagnosis of GCA. In particular, a vascular smooth, linear pattern with FDG uptake more intense than that of the liver is considered highly specific for vasculitis (**Fig. 4**).[45] PET has also proved useful in the early diagnosis of TAK. In 5 patients with early, clinically active TAK, high FDG uptake was observed in all patients and in 76% of vascular segments.[46] In another study, PET was 75% sensitive and 65% specific in identifying patients with active TAK.[47] The impact of PET on the diagnosis of LVV has recently been formally assessed in a study in which an international experts' panel was asked to determine diagnoses and clinical management in patients with suspected LVV with and without having access to the results of PET, respectively.[48] PET had an overall sensitivity of 73%, a specificity of 84%, a positive predictive value of 82%, and a negative predictive value of 77%, and the addition of PET increased the diagnostic accuracy from 54% to 71%. These findings thus provide evidence that PET significantly increases the overall diagnostic accuracy in a significant proportion of patients with suspected LVV. PET has only a modest to fair correlation with clinical assessment of LVV,[47,49] which may be accounted for, at least in part, by the unsatisfactory specificity and sensitivity of current clinimetric assessment tools of LVV.[50,51] On the other hand, the diagnostic accuracy of PET has been shown to dramatically decline (by nearly 50%) after the institution of GC or immunosuppressive treatment.[48] In terms of prognostic value, high vascular FDG uptake has been shown to predict the development of thoracic, but not aortic, aneurysms in patients with GCA.[52]

A distinctive advantage of PET is its ability to visualize almost all large vessels except the renal arteries and TA. Limitations of PET are its limited availability, its high costs, and the inability to provide anatomic details of the vessel wall and lumen.[3] PET involves only a small dose of radiation.[3]

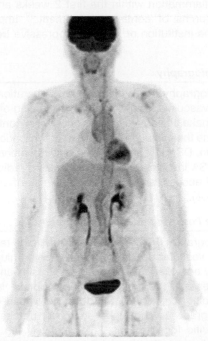

Fig. 4. PET coronal view showing increased (grade 3 on a 0–3 scale) ^{18}F-FDG uptake by the thoracic and abdominal aorta as well as by the iliac, femoral, common carotid arteries bilaterally, and by the right subclavian and axillary arteries in a patient with GCA involving large vessels.

CP

CP is a rare disease characterized by a fibroinflammatory reaction spreading from the aorta into the retroperitoneum, which can present as idiopathic retroperitoneal fibrosis, inflammatory abdominal aortic aneurysm, or perianeurysmal retroperitoneal fibrosis.[53] In a study from our group of 7 patients with CP,[54] PET showed active vasculitis of the abdominal aorta, of the iliac arteries, or both, in all patients with CP but not in matched controls (**Fig. 5**). Another half of patients also had involvement of other large vessels. These findings strongly argue for a vasculitic nature of CP.[55] Abdominal CT and MR can disclose signs of active aortitis (vessel wall thickening with mural enhancement) as well as visualize the periaortic tissue, whereas CTA and MRA are useful to screen for aortic dilation (**Fig. 6**).[55]

PCNSV

PCNSV is a vasculitis affecting the brain and rarely the spinal cord.[56,57] PCNSV is usually classified according to the criteria proposed by Calabrese, which comprise the history or presence of an acquired neurologic deficit, histologic or angiographic evidence of vasculitis, and no evidence of systemic vasculitis or other condition that could cause the angiographic or pathologic features.[58] Histologic confirmation of vasculitis is required for a definite diagnosis, but a probable diagnosis can be made if there are characteristic angiographic lesions associated with MR and cerebrospinal fluid changes consistent with PCNSV.[59] MR is the key screening test for PCNSV, because its sensitivity is close to 100%,[60] whereas CT is notoriously insensitive in picking up the subtle secondary signs of vasculitis (ie, infarct and ischemia).[61]

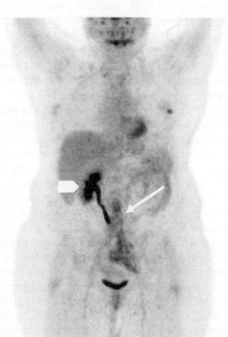

Fig. 5. PET coronal view of a patient with CP (retroperitoneal fibrosis) showing heterogeneous ^{18}F-FDG uptake around the abdominal aorta (*arrow*) spreading caudally to the iliac arteries. Note the concomitant urine retention in the right calyx (*arrowhead*) and the poor visualization of the left kidney, suggestive of hydronephrosis.

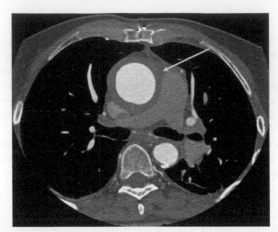

Fig. 6. CTA, axial view of the ascending aorta of a patient with retroperitoneal fibrosis. Note the conspicuous thickening of the aortic wall (*arrow*). (*Courtesy of* Dr Lucia Spaggiari, MD, Radiology Department, Arcispedale Santa Maria Nuova, Reggio Emilia, Italy.)

However, MR changes are largely nonspecific. In a retrospective review, in 85% of cases, MR showed multiple bilateral ischemic lesions, in 63% lesions in both the cortex and the white matter, in one-third leptomeningeal enhancement, and occasionally (10%) intracranial hemorrhage.[56] Perivascular enhancement is a specific, but unusual, sign of this type of vasculitis.[62] PET is of limited usefulness for PCNSV because of background increased FDG uptake by the brain parenchyma and the lack of resolution of vessels smaller than 4 mm.[63,64] In contrast, a new tracer known as [11C]PK11195, which preferentially binds to the peripheral benzodiazepine binding site of activated macrophages, holds promise for use in PCNSV, because macrophages are predominant along the vessel wall in areas of vascular inflammation.[61,65] Therefore, nuclear studies using [11C]PK11195 could theoretically help clarify cases in which MR findings are ambiguous.

An abnormal MR study of the central nervous system (CNS) must be complemented by angiography. DSA has a sensitivity of 40% to 90% and specificity of 30% for PCNSV.[60] Changes highly suggestive of vasculitis are alternating areas of smooth-wall narrowing and dilatation (rarely aneurysms) of cerebral arteries or arterial occlusions affecting many cerebral vessels in the absence of proximal vascular atherosclerosis or other recognized abnormalities. In contrast, single abnormalities in several arteries or several abnormalities in 1 artery are less consistent with PCNSV (**Fig. 7**).[66] MRA is approximately 20% less sensitive than DSA to detect vessel abnormalities in PCNSV.[66] If angiographic studies are negative or not typical and clinical findings are in question, brain biopsy is advised to secure the diagnosis. Imaging studies are also helpful to define the prognosis of PCNSV. In this regard, there is evidence that PCNSV characterized by small-vessel involvement (ie, a negative angiography and a positive biopsy) has a better outcome.[67] Similarly, prominent leptomeningeal enhancement on MR has been mapped to a subtype of PCNSV with small leptomeningeal artery vasculitis and a favorable response to therapy.[68] Rapidly progressive PCNSV represents the worst end of the clinical spectrum of this vasculitis.[69] These patients have a rapidly progressive course, with often fatal outcome. They present with bilateral, multiple, large cerebral vessel lesions on angiograms and multiple bilateral cerebral infarctions. These patients respond poorly to traditional immunosuppressive treatment.

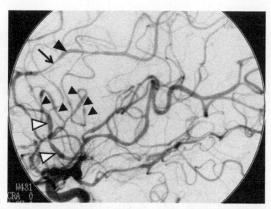

Fig. 7. DSA. (*Right*) Anterior cerebral artery is intermittently dilated (*white arrowheads*). The proximal aspect of pericallosal artery is narrowed (*black arrow*) and its distal aspect is dilated (*black arrowhead*). Multiple segmental stenosis and enlargements are also identified in the middle cerebral artery branches (*small black arrowheads*). (*Courtesy of* Dr John Huston III, MD, Department of Radiology, Mayo Clinic, Rochester, MN.)

ADAMANTIADES-BEHÇET DISEASE

Adamantiades-Behçet disease (ABD) is a PSV that may affect arteries and veins of any caliber. Imaging studies are required to investigate ABD-related CNS and large-vessel manifestations. CNS involvement in ABD is typically characterized by an aseptic meningoencephalitis (neuro-Behçet disease) with prevalent involvement of the brainstem, basal ganglia, and deep hemispheric white matter; however, a few patients present with intracranial hypertension caused by vascular disease.[70] Less common presentations of neuro-Behçet disease include periventricular parenchymal lesions mimicking multiple sclerosis,[71] a tumorlike single mass,[72] and optic neuropathy.[73] Parenchymal lesions are isointense to hypointense on T1-weighted and hyperintense on T2-weighted and fluid-attenuated inversion recovery (FLAIR) sequences (**Fig. 8**),[70] whereas occlusion of dural sinuses is typically noted in patients with intracranial hypertension.[74] In patients with optic neuropathy, the only sign on MR may be optic nerve enhancement,[73] which is usually subtle and may sometimes be absent despite active neuropathy (personal observations). Active lesions usually markedly regress or resolve after successful therapy, although chronic sequelae may be observed.[74]

Vascular involvement in ABD can manifest as thromboses, stenoses, occlusions, and aneurysms.[75] The most common manifestation is superficial or deep vein thrombosis, mainly of the lower limbs.[76] However, the most dreaded complication of vascular Behçet disease is the development of aneurysms of the pulmonary artery, a rare (less than 5% of all patients with ABD) manifestation that occurs most often in young males and carries a high risk of rupture. Helical CT is considered the technique of choice to document pulmonary aneurysms.[77]

KD

KD is an acute, self-limiting vasculitis of infants and young children.[78] KD is characterized by fever, bilateral conjunctivitis, erythema of the lips and oral mucosa, rash, and cervical lymphadenopathy. Coronary artery aneurysms or ectasia develop in approximately 20% of untreated children. Coronary angiography has traditionally been used to diagnose coronary artery alterations, but has now largely been superseded by

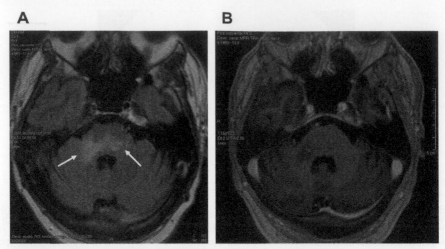

Fig. 8. MR (FLAIR) (*A*) and multiplanar reformation (*B*) images showing hyperintense punctate lesions (*arrows*) at the border between pons and right peduncle in a patient with active neuro-Behçet disease. (*Courtesy of* Dr Lucia Spaggiari, MD, Radiology Department, Arcispedale Santa Maria Nuova, Reggio Emilia, Italy.)

echocardiography, which has been shown to have both high sensitivity (95%) and specificity (99%) compared with angiography without incurring exposure to radiation.[79] The American Heart Association recommends that patients with KD should be evaluated by echocardiography at presentation, at 2 weeks, and after 6 to 8 weeks.[78] Because myocarditis and depressed ventricular contractility may also occur early on in KD, left ventricular function also ought to be assessed.[78] MRA is an acceptable alternative to angiography when transthoracic echocardiography image quality is unsatisfactory.[78,80]

PAN

PAN is a medium-vessel necrotizing vasculitis with predominant renal (70%–80% of cases) and gastrointestinal, peripheral nerve system, or cutaneous involvement (~50% of cases).[81] Characteristic angiographic findings of PAN are multiple small aneurysms, although vessel occlusions leading to infarctions may also occur, often in association with aneurysms.[81] The presence of numerous (>30) aneurysms is considered almost diagnostic for PAN.[82] The mesenteric artery, the upper limb vessels, the renal arteries, and the hepatic artery are affected in more than two-thirds of patients.[81] Regression of vascular lesions after therapy has been reported.[83] Imaging is helpful to differentiate PAN from other disorders causing aneurysms, particularly fibromuscular dysplasia and mycotic infection. In fibromuscular dysplasia, aneurysms are irregular and often have a string-of-beads appearance on angiography caused by alternating areas of stenosis and aneurysms, whereas mycotic aneurysms are less numerous than those seen in PAN.[81]

AAV

AVV comprise granulomatosis with polyangiitis (GPA, formerly known as Wegener granulomatosis), Churg-Strauss syndrome (CSS) and microscopic polyangiitis (MPA). Imaging studies are usually required to document involvement of internal organs, especially of the lung, which is commonly affected in all AAV.

Pulmonary Imaging

About 50% to 80% of patients with GPA have pulmonary involvement.[84] Chest radiography often reveals bilateral, reticular, or nodular opacities. However, chest CT is needed to better define lung lesions. In a series of 57 patients, CT revealed predominantly subpleural or diffuse nodules or masses in 89% patients (bilateral in 70%), with 22% of nodules or masses showing cavitation and 6% spiculation.[85] Areas of predominantly subpleural consolidation were observed in 30%, mimicking pulmonary infarction in 71% of patients. Twenty-six percent of patients had evidence of patchy ground-glass attenuation (GGA), whereas bronchial wall thickening was observed in 56%. Less common findings included pleural effusion and lymphadenopathy.

Nearly all patients with CSS have respiratory symptoms, especially asthma.[84] Chest radiography may reveal recurrent pulmonary infiltrates mainly localized to the lower lobes and, less frequently, reticulonodular opacities, bronchial wall thickening, and multiple nodules.[86] High-resolution chest CT typically shows bilateral patchy GGA with predominant subpleural and lower lobe distribution or areas of consolidation, but centrilobular nodules, bronchial wall thickening, increased vessel caliber, lymphadenopathy, hyperinflation, and serosal effusions may also be observed.[86] Pulmonary infiltrates may reflect either eosinophilic infiltrates or vasculitic lesions.[86] Some findings, such as hyperinflation and bronchial wall thickening, are likely to be related to asthma.

About 20% to 60% of patients with MPA have evidence of pulmonary involvement, usually diffuse alveolar hemorrhage.[84] In patients with alveolar hemorrhage, chest radiographs show diffuse, bilateral, alveolar infiltrates, whereas CT shows widespread GGA.[87,88] Interstitial lung disease has also occasionally been linked to MPA.[89]

CNS Imaging

Involvement of the CNS in AAV is rare (0%–8% of patients), but not exceptional. Brain MR typically shows multiple ischemic (sometimes hemorrhagic) lesions, mainly affecting the white matter.[90] Angiography is usually negative, because the diameter of the arteries affected is below the power of resolution of angiography.[90]

Imaging of Other Organs

The nose and cranial sinuses are often affected by GPA. MR or CT can disclose sinus mucosal edema and thickening, bony destruction, and erosions of surrounding structures. Involvement of abdominal organs, often ischemic in nature, can also occur.[91] CT of the abdomen is useful to show both vasculitic organ involvement and complications such as gastrointestinal perforation secondary to vasculitis.[92]

SUMMARY

Imaging studies are useful to document TA inflammation in GCA and essential to show large-vessel inflammation in early LVV, when vascular lesions have often not yet developed and clinical examination may thus be unrevealing. On the other hand, in established LVV, imaging studies are more sensitive than clinical examination and can therefore significantly increase the diagnostic accuracy or the capacity to disclose vascular complications.[93] However, imaging findings can be affected by immunosuppressive treatment. Furthermore, imaging has only a limited capacity to predict the development of new vascular lesions.

A major caveat in interpreting vascular imaging findings is the need to differentiate vasculitis from atherosclerosis. The presence of long, smooth stenoses that symmetrically affect the vessel wall, a marked increase in vessel wall thickening on morphologic imaging,[94] or high-intensity vascular FDG uptake on PET[3] point to vasculitis over atherosclerosis. In contrast, asymmetric, patchy lesions, particularly if associated with calcifications, suggest atherosclerosis.[3] In medium-vessel vasculitis, alternative, less hazardous techniques may often obviate resorting to conventional angiography. The wide array of imaging techniques available is a key support to the clinician in diagnosing vasculitis and will most likely play an ever more important role in the future.

REFERENCES

1. Scott DG, Watts RA. Classification and epidemiology of systemic vasculitis. Br J Rheumatol 1994;33:897–9.
2. Grayson PC, Maksimowicz-McKinnon K, Clark TM, et al. Distribution of arterial lesions in Takayasu's arteritis and giant cell arteritis. Ann Rheum Dis 2012;71: 1329–34.
3. Pipitone N, Versari A, Salvarani C. Role of imaging studies in the diagnosis and follow-up of large-vessel vasculitis: an update. Rheumatology (Oxford) 2008;47: 403–8.
4. Schmidt WA, Kraft HE, Vorpahl K, et al. Color duplex ultrasonography in the diagnosis of temporal arteritis. N Engl J Med 1997;337:1336–42.
5. Ball EL, Walsh SR, Tang TY, et al. Role of ultrasonography in the diagnosis of temporal arteritis. Br J Surg 2010;97:1765–71.
6. Arida A, Kyprianou M, Kanakis M, et al. The diagnostic value of ultrasonography-derived edema of the temporal artery wall in giant cell arteritis: a second meta-analysis. BMC Musculoskelet Disord 2010;11:44.
7. Schmidt WA, Krause A, Schicke B, et al. Do temporal artery duplex ultrasound findings correlate with ophthalmic complications in giant cell arteritis? Rheumatology (Oxford) 2009;48:383–5.
8. Schmidt WA, Natusch A, Moller DE, et al. Involvement of peripheral arteries in giant cell arteritis: a color Doppler sonography study. Clin Exp Rheumatol 2002;20:309–18.
9. Aschwanden M, Kesten F, Stern M, et al. Vascular involvement in patients with giant cell arteritis determined by duplex sonography of 2x11 arterial regions. Ann Rheum Dis 2010;69:1356–9.
10. Ghinoi A, Pipitone N, Nicolini A, et al. Large-vessel involvement in recent-onset giant cell arteritis: a case-control colour-Doppler sonography study. Rheumatology (Oxford) 2012;51:730–4.
11. Schmidt WA, Seifert A, Gromnica-Ihle E, et al. Ultrasound of proximal upper extremity arteries to increase the diagnostic yield in large-vessel giant cell arteritis. Rheumatology (Oxford) 2008;47:96–101.
12. Bossert M, Prati C, Balblanc JC, et al. Aortic involvement in giant cell arteritis: current data. Joint Bone Spine 2011;78:246–51.
13. Maeda H, Handa N, Matsumoto M, et al. Carotid lesions detected by B-mode ultrasonography in Takayasu's arteritis: "macaroni sign" as an indicator of the disease. Ultrasound Med Biol 1991;17:695–701.
14. Nicoletti G, Mannarella C, Nigro A, et al. The "macaroni sign" of Takayasu's arteritis. J Rheumatol 2009;36:2042–3.
15. Taniguchi N, Itoh K, Honda M, et al. Comparative ultrasonographic and angiographic study of carotid arterial lesions in Takayasu's arteritis. Angiology 1997; 48:9–20.

16. Giordana P, Baque-Juston MC, Jeandel PY, et al. Contrast-enhanced ultrasound of carotid artery wall in Takayasu disease: first evidence of application in diagnosis and monitoring of response to treatment. Circulation 2011;124:245–7.

17. Magnoni M, Dagna L, Coli S, et al. Assessment of Takayasu arteritis activity by carotid contrast-enhanced ultrasound. Circ Cardiovasc Imaging 2011;4:e1–2.

18. De Miguel ME, Roxo A, Castillo C, et al. The utility and sensitivity of colour Doppler ultrasound in monitoring changes in giant cell arteritis. Clin Exp Rheumatol 2012;30:S34–8.

19. Schmidt WA, Nerenheim A, Seipelt E, et al. Diagnosis of early Takayasu arteritis with sonography. Rheumatology (Oxford) 2002;41:496–502.

20. Hauenstein C, Reinhard M, Geiger J, et al. Effects of early corticosteroid treatment on magnetic resonance imaging and ultrasonography findings in giant cell arteritis. Rheumatology (Oxford) 2012;51:1999–2003.

21. Kissin EY, Merkel PA. Diagnostic imaging in Takayasu arteritis. Curr Opin Rheumatol 2004;16:31–7.

22. De ME, Castillo C, Rodriguez A, et al. Learning and reliability of colour Doppler ultrasound in giant cell arteritis. Clin Exp Rheumatol 2009;27:S53–8.

23. Gotway MB, Araoz PA, Macedo TA, et al. Imaging findings in Takayasu's arteritis. AJR Am J Roentgenol 2005;184:1945–50.

24. Yoshida S, Akiba H, Tamakawa M, et al. The spectrum of findings in supra-aortic Takayasu's arteritis as seen on spiral CT angiography and digital subtraction angiography. Cardiovasc Intervent Radiol 2001;24:117–21.

25. Chung JW, Kim HC, Choi YH, et al. Patterns of aortic involvement in Takayasu arteritis and its clinical implications: evaluation with spiral computed tomography angiography. J Vasc Surg 2007;45:906–14.

26. Paul JF, Fiessinger JN, Sapoval M, et al. Follow-up electron beam CT for the management of early phase Takayasu arteritis. J Comput Assist Tomogr 2001; 25:924–31.

27. Yamada I, Nakagawa T, Himeno Y, et al. Takayasu arteritis: evaluation of the thoracic aorta with CT angiography. Radiology 1998;209:103–9.

28. Prieto-Gonzalez S, Arguis P, Garcia-Martinez A, et al. Large vessel involvement in biopsy-proven giant cell arteritis: prospective study in 40 newly diagnosed patients using CT angiography. Ann Rheum Dis 2012;71:1170–6.

29. Choe YH, Kim DK, Koh EM, et al. Takayasu arteritis: diagnosis with MR imaging and MR angiography in acute and chronic active stages. J Magn Reson Imaging 1999;10:751–7.

30. Choe YH, Lee WR. Magnetic resonance imaging diagnosis of Takayasu arteritis. Int J Cardiol 1998;66(Suppl 1):S175–9.

31. Geiger J, Bley T, Uhl M, et al. Diagnostic value of T2-weighted imaging for the detection of superficial cranial artery inflammation in giant cell arteritis. J Magn Reson Imaging 2010;31:470–4.

32. Ghinoi A, Zuccoli G, Nicolini A, et al. 1T magnetic resonance imaging in the diagnosis of giant cell arteritis: comparison with ultrasonography and physical examination of temporal arteries. Clin Exp Rheumatol 2008;26:S76–80.

33. Bley TA, Uhl M, Carew J, et al. Diagnostic value of high-resolution MR imaging in giant cell arteritis. AJNR Am J Neuroradiol 2007;28:1722–7.

34. Brack A, Martinez-Taboada V, Stanson A, et al. Disease pattern in cranial and large-vessel giant cell arteritis. Arthritis Rheum 1999;42:311–7.

35. Angeli E, Vanzulli A, Venturini M, et al. The role of radiology in the diagnosis and management of Takayasu's arteritis. J Nephrol 2001;14:514–24.

36. Garg SK, Mohan S, Kumar S. Diagnostic value of 3D contrast-enhanced magnetic resonance angiography in Takayasu's arteritis–a comparative study with digital subtraction angiography. Eur Radiol 2011;21:1658–66.
37. Tso E, Flamm SD, White RD, et al. Takayasu arteritis: utility and limitations of magnetic resonance imaging in diagnosis and treatment. Arthritis Rheum 2002; 46:1634–42.
38. Bley TA, Markl M, Schelp M, et al. Mural inflammatory hyperenhancement in MRI of giant cell (temporal) arteritis resolves under corticosteroid treatment. Rheumatology (Oxford) 2008;47:65–7.
39. Bley TA, Ness T, Warnatz K, et al. Influence of corticosteroid treatment on MRI findings in giant cell arteritis. Clin Rheumatol 2007;26:1541–3.
40. Ahdab R, Thabuy F, Menager de FE, et al. Reversible vertebral artery stenosis following corticotherapy in giant cell arteritis. Eur Neurol 2008;59:331.
41. Willinsky RA, Taylor SM, TerBrugge K, et al. Neurologic complications of cerebral angiography: prospective analysis of 2,899 procedures and review of the literature. Radiology 2003;227:522–8.
42. Meller J, Strutz F, Siefker U, et al. Early diagnosis and follow-up of aortitis with [(18)F]FDG PET and MRI. Eur J Nucl Med Mol Imaging 2003;30:730–6.
43. Belhocine T, Blockmans D, Hustinx R, et al. Imaging of large vessel vasculitis with (18)FDG PET: illusion or reality? A critical review of the literature data. Eur J Nucl Med Mol Imaging 2003;30:1305–13.
44. Hautzel H, Sander O, Heinzel A, et al. Assessment of large-vessel involvement in giant cell arteritis with 18F-FDG PET: introducing an ROC-analysis-based cutoff ratio. J Nucl Med 2008;49:1107–13.
45. Besson FL, Parienti JJ, Bienvenu B, et al. Diagnostic performance of (1)(8)F-fluorodeoxyglucose positron emission tomography in giant cell arteritis: a systematic review and meta-analysis. Eur J Nucl Med Mol Imaging 2011;38:1764–72.
46. Meller J, Grabbe E, Becker W, et al. Value of F-18 FDG hybrid camera PET and MRI in early Takayasu aortitis. Eur Radiol 2003;13:400–5.
47. Lee KH, Cho A, Choi YJ, et al. The role of (18) F-fluorodeoxyglucose-positron emission tomography in the assessment of disease activity in patients with Takayasu arteritis. Arthritis Rheum 2012;64:866–75.
48. Fuchs M, Briel M, Daikeler T, et al. The impact of 18F-FDG PET on the management of patients with suspected large vessel vasculitis. Eur J Nucl Med Mol Imaging 2012;39:344–53.
49. Arnaud L, Haroche J, Malek Z, et al. Is (18)F-fluorodeoxyglucose positron emission tomography scanning a reliable way to assess disease activity in Takayasu arteritis? Arthritis Rheum 2009;60:1193–200.
50. Kerr GS, Hallahan CW, Giordano J, et al. Takayasu arteritis. Ann Intern Med 1994; 120:919–29.
51. Aydin SZ, Yilmaz N, Akar S, et al. Assessment of disease activity and progression in Takayasu's arteritis with Disease Extent Index-Takayasu. Rheumatology (Oxford) 2010;49:1889–93.
52. Blockmans D, Coudyzer W, Vanderschueren S, et al. Relationship between fluorodeoxyglucose uptake in the large vessels and late aortic diameter in giant cell arteritis. Rheumatology (Oxford) 2008;47:1179–84.
53. Vaglio A, Salvarani C, Buzio C. Retroperitoneal fibrosis. Lancet 2006;367:241–51.
54. Salvarani C, Pipitone N, Versari A, et al. Positron emission tomography (PET): evaluation of chronic periaortitis. Arthritis Rheum 2005;53:298–303.
55. Vaglio A, Pipitone N, Salvarani C. Chronic periaortitis: a large-vessel vasculitis? Curr Opin Rheumatol 2011;23:1–6.

56. Salvarani C, Brown RD Jr, Calamia KT, et al. Primary central nervous system vasculitis: analysis of 101 patients. Ann Neurol 2007;62:442–51.
57. Salvarani C, Brown RD Jr, Calamia KT, et al. Primary CNS vasculitis with spinal cord involvement. Neurology 2008;70:2394–400.
58. Calabrese LH, Mallek JA. Primary angiitis of the central nervous system. Report of 8 new cases, review of the literature, and proposal for diagnostic criteria. Medicine (Baltimore) 1988;67:20–39.
59. Birnbaum J, Hellmann DB. Primary angiitis of the central nervous system. Arch Neurol 2009;66:704–9.
60. Salvarani C, Brown RD Jr, Hunder GG. Adult primary central nervous system vasculitis: an update. Curr Opin Rheumatol 2012;24:46–52.
61. Zuccoli G, Pipitone N, Haldipur A, et al. Imaging findings in primary central nervous system vasculitis. Clin Exp Rheumatol 2011;29:S104–9.
62. Salvarani C, Brown RD Jr, Huston J III, et al. Prominent perivascular enhancement in primary central nervous system vasculitis. Clin Exp Rheumatol 2008; 26:S111.
63. Gomes LJ. The role of imaging in the diagnosis of central nervous system vasculitis. Curr Allergy Asthma Rep 2010;10:163–70.
64. Blockmans D, Bley T, Schmidt W. Imaging for large-vessel vasculitis. Curr Opin Rheumatol 2009;21:19–28.
65. Pugliese F, Gaemperli O, Kinderlerer AR, et al. Imaging of vascular inflammation with [11C]-PK11195 and positron emission tomography/computed tomography angiography. J Am Coll Cardiol 2010;56:653–61.
66. Salvarani C, Brown RD Jr, Hunder GG. Adult primary central nervous system vasculitis. Lancet 2012;380:767–77.
67. Salvarani C, Brown RD Jr, Calamia KT, et al. Angiography-negative primary central nervous system vasculitis: a syndrome involving small cerebral vessels. Medicine (Baltimore) 2008;87:264–71.
68. Salvarani C, Brown RD Jr, Calamia KT, et al. Primary central nervous system vasculitis with prominent leptomeningeal enhancement: a subset with a benign outcome. Arthritis Rheum 2008;58:595–603.
69. Salvarani C, Brown RD Jr, Calamia KT, et al. Rapidly progressive primary central nervous system vasculitis. Rheumatology (Oxford) 2011;50:349–58.
70. Akman-Demir G, Bahar S, Coban O, et al. Cranial MRI in Behcet's disease: 134 examinations of 98 patients. Neuroradiology 2003;45:851–9.
71. Serdaroglu P. Behcet's disease and the nervous system. J Neurol 1998;245: 197–205.
72. Noel N, Hutie M, Wechsler B, et al. Pseudotumoural presentation of neuro-Behcet's disease: case series and review of literature. Rheumatology (Oxford) 2012;51:1216–25.
73. Kocer N, Islak C, Siva A, et al. CNS involvement in neuro-Behcet syndrome: an MR study. AJNR Am J Neuroradiol 1999;20:1015–24.
74. Akman-Demir G, Serdaroglu P, Tasci B. Clinical patterns of neurological involvement in Behcet's disease: evaluation of 200 patients. The Neuro-Behcet Study Group. Brain 1999;122(Pt 11):2171–82.
75. Calamia KT, Schirmer M, Melikoglu M. Major vessel involvement in Behcet's disease: an update. Curr Opin Rheumatol 2011;23:24–31.
76. Duzgun N, Ates A, Aydintug OT, et al. Characteristics of vascular involvement in Behcet's disease. Scand J Rheumatol 2006;35:65–8.
77. Erkan F. Pulmonary involvement in Behcet disease. Curr Opin Pulm Med 1999;5: 314–8.

78. Newburger JW, Takahashi M, Gerber MA, et al. Diagnosis, treatment, and long-term management of Kawasaki disease: a statement for health professionals from the Committee on Rheumatic Fever, Endocarditis and Kawasaki Disease, Council on Cardiovascular Disease in the Young, American Heart Association. Circulation 2004;110:2747–71.
79. Hiraishi S, Misawa H, Takeda N, et al. Transthoracic ultrasonic visualisation of coronary aneurysm, stenosis, and occlusion in Kawasaki disease. Heart 2000; 83:400–5.
80. Greil GF, Stuber M, Botnar RM, et al. Coronary magnetic resonance angiography in adolescents and young adults with Kawasaki disease. Circulation 2002;105: 908–11.
81. Stanson AW, Friese JL, Johnson CM, et al. Polyarteritis nodosa: spectrum of angiographic findings. Radiographics 2001;21:151–9.
82. Hekali P, Kajander H, Pajari R, et al. Diagnostic significance of angiographically observed visceral aneurysms with regard to polyarteritis nodosa. Acta Radiol 1991;32:143–8.
83. Tarhan NC, Coskun M, Kayahan EM, et al. Regression of abdominal visceral aneurysms in polyarteritis nodosa: CT findings. AJR Am J Roentgenol 2003; 180:1617–9.
84. Puechal X. Antineutrophil cytoplasmic antibody-associated vasculitides. Joint Bone Spine 2007;74:427–35.
85. Lohrmann C, Uhl M, Kotter E, et al. Pulmonary manifestations of Wegener granulomatosis: CT findings in 57 patients and a review of the literature. Eur J Radiol 2005;53:471–7.
86. Choi YH, Im JG, Han BK, et al. Thoracic manifestation of Churg-Strauss syndrome: radiologic and clinical findings. Chest 2000;117:117–24.
87. Seo JB, Im JG, Chung JW, et al. Pulmonary vasculitis: the spectrum of radiological findings. Br J Radiol 2000;73:1224–31.
88. Lauque D, Cadranel J, Lazor R, et al. Microscopic polyangiitis with alveolar hemorrhage. A study of 29 cases and review of the literature. Groupe d'Etudes et de Recherche sur les Maladies "Orphelines" Pulmonaires (GERM"O"P). Medicine (Baltimore) 2000;79:222–33.
89. Gomez-Puerta JA, Espinosa G, Morla R, et al. Interstitial lung disease as a presenting manifestation of microscopic polyangiitis successfully treated with mycophenolate mofetil. Clin Exp Rheumatol 2009;27:166–7.
90. Ghinoi A, Zuccoli G, Pipitone N, et al. Anti-neutrophil cytoplasmic antibody (ANCA)-associated vasculitis involving the central nervous system: case report and review of the literature. Clin Exp Rheumatol 2010;28:759–66.
91. Ghinoi A, Pipitone N, Cavazza A, et al. Wegener granulomatosis with spleen infarction: case report and review of the literature. Semin Arthritis Rheum 2008; 37:328–33.
92. Deniz K, Ozseker HS, Balas S, et al. Intestinal involvement in Wegener's granulomatosis. J Gastrointestin Liver Dis 2007;16:329–31.
93. Grayson PC, Tomasson G, Cuthbertson D, et al. Association of vascular physical examination findings and arteriographic lesions in large vessel vasculitis. J Rheumatol 2012;39:303–9.
94. Arnaud L, Haroche J, Amoura Z. The presence of atherosclerotic plaques in patients with Takayasu arteritis: comment on the article by Keenan et al. Arthritis Rheum 2010;62:1558–9.

Imaging of Osteoporosis

Robert Schneider, MD

KEYWORDS

- Osteoporosis • Bone density • Bone densitometry • Absorptiometry
- Bone architecture • Insufficiency fractures

KEY POINTS

- Several routine imaging modalities are used for evaluation of bone strength, including radiography, CT, MRI, absorptiometry, and quantitative ultrasound densitometry (QUS).
- Detection of atraumatic fractures is important for the detection of decreased bone strength.
- Dual-energy x-ray absorptiometry (DXA) is the standard method for measuring bone density and is used in the World Health Organization (WHO) classification of osteoporosis.
- Advanced imaging techniques using CT, MRI, DXA, and computerized analysis are providing increased information about bone architecture and bone strength.

INTRODUCTION

Various imaging techniques are used for evaluating bone density and bone quality. Bone strength is ultimately defined by a combination of bone density and bone quality. Bone quality is a reflection of its component parts, including bone architecture, bone turnover, mineralization, and microfractures.[1] Bone density is a term referring to the amount of mineral matter per volume of bones and accounts for approximately 60% of bone strength.[2] Routinely used imaging modalities, such as radiography, CT, MRI, and DXA, and advanced techniques, which use high-resolution CT and MRI, and computerized quantitative methodology are used to study osteoporosis and bone strength.[3–6] The advanced laboratory and imaging techniques are used mainly in experimental studies in humans and laboratory animals.[7,8] As stated by Griffith and Genant,[3] limitations of these advanced techniques include cost, the fact that they are not widely available, their requirement for technical expertise that is limited, and the need for biopsy specimens; all hinder their adoption into mainstream clinical practice. Mainstream techniques and their interpretation are improving, often driven by the improvements in therapy.

Department of Radiology and Imaging, Hospital for Special Surgery, 535 East 70th Street, New York, NY 10021, USA
E-mail address: Schneiderr@hss.edu

Rheum Dis Clin N Am 39 (2013) 609–631
http://dx.doi.org/10.1016/j.rdc.2013.02.016
0889-857X/13/$ – see front matter © 2013 Elsevier Inc. All rights reserved.

Rheumatic diseases are often associated with osteoporosis.[9] Drug therapy, especially corticosteroids, may cause bone loss. Disease and pain in the joints cause decreased mobility, leading to disuse osteoporosis. The disease processes themselves may release proinflammatory cytokines that lead to resorption of bone.[7,8] The presence of rheumatologic disease should lead to evaluation of bone density earlier than in the otherwise normal population, and there are treatments of diseases, such as rheumatoid arthritis, that control both the disease and the attendant bone loss and risk of fracture.[10]

Osteoporosis itself does not cause pain and is clinically silent except for fracture. Atraumatic or low-impact/fragility fractures are associated with osteoporosis. Vertebral body, femoral neck, or intertrochanteric region of the femur and distal radius are frequent sites of these fractures. If compression fracture of the spine is present, without causal trauma, tumor, or infection, patients can be classified as having osteoporosis, regardless of bone density measurements (**Fig. 1**). These fractures may cause an accentuation of the thoraic kyphosis. Insufficiency fractures are stress fractures that occur with normal stress on abnormal bone. They often occur in the metaphyses of long bones, pubis and ischium, and femoral neck (**Fig. 2**). Detection of these fractures may be delayed after the onset of symptoms; thus, imaging methods are crucial for diagnosis of these fractures, with MRI, radionuclide bone scanning, and positron emission tomography (PET) more sensitive than radiography.

DXA is the standard method for evaluating bone density in clinical practice. Many other methods are also available but less frequently used.[11] Although there is a good correlation between bone density and fracture risk, fractures cannot always be predicted by bone density measurements alone.[12,13]

The gold standard for evaluating bone density and bone architecture has been considered bone biopsy with histologic analysis of undecalcified specimens with histomorphometry.[14,15] Tetracycline labeling with histomorphometry helps evaluate bone

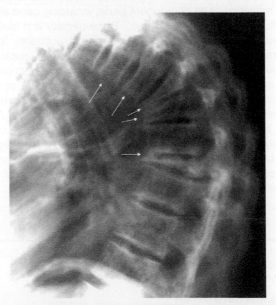

Fig. 1. Osteoporotic compression fractures of the thoracic spine (*arrows*) and accentuation of the thoracic kyphosis.

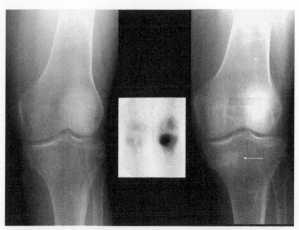

Fig. 2. Insufficiency fracture of the metaphysis of the left tibia. The initial radiograph was normal. The bone scan at the same time showed high uptake in the medial tibia. On the radiograph at 3 weeks, there is sclerosis in the medial metaphysis of the tibia (*arrow*).

turnover. The requirement for biopsy specimens makes it impractical for routine clinical use. Bone biopsy with histomorphometry is usually not necessary for diagnosis of osteoporosis but may be helpful in cases where the cause of increased fragility is uncertain, as in osteomalacia and renal osteodystrophy.[16,17] Because bone biopsy is not practical for screening or evaluating large numbers of patients, noninvasive imaging methods are used most frequently.

QUALITATIVE IMAGING

After history and physical examination, radiographs are usually the initial imaging modality. Radiographs evaluate bone density by assessing radiolucency, trabecular architecture, and cortical thickness. There is information on standard radiographs that can help evaluate bone density and structure.[18] The ability to judge bone density by assessing radiolucency is limited by variations in radiographic technique, settings for contrast on digital radiography and picture archiving communication systems, and size of patient and overlying soft tissues. Approximately 30% to 80% or more of bone must be lost on radiographs of the spine before it can be reliably detected.[19] In osteoporosis, the horizontal trabeculae in the spine are resorbed, leading to a prominent appearance of the remaining vertical trabeculae. The subchondral cortices of the end plates in the spine and at the articular surfaces of the bones around the joint become prominent because of the greater resorption of the cancellous bone beneath them. The bone architecture may be better seen on CT (**Fig. 3**). Joint inflammation and high turnover of cancellous bone help explain periarticular osteoporosis found in inflammatory arthritis (**Fig. 4**). Osteoporosis around the articular surfaces may simulate bony erosions. In osteoporosis, the cortex remains intact, although it may be difficult to see because of thinning. Cortical thinning, endosteal scaloping, and alteration of trabecular pattern are radiographic findings in osteoporosis that can be visually detected on radiographs. Endosteal scalloping from resorption can be difficult to differentiate from metastatic disease or myeloma.

Visual (qualitative) assessment of radiographs is the most commonly used method for diagnosis of spine fractures in clinical practice. The lateral view of a chest radiograph should be carefully assessed for compression fractures, because these

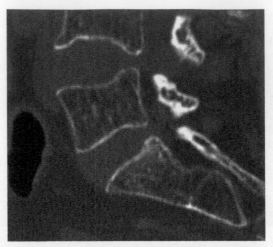

Fig. 3. Osteoporosis, with loss of horizontal trabeculae in the vertebral body and accentuation of the vertical, and end plate deformities on sagittal CT image.

fractures are often overlooked or not reported (**Fig. 5**). In a study of emergency room patients over 60 years of age who had chest radiographs, Majumdar and colleagues[20] reported that 16% had moderate or severe compression fractures and only 40% were reported. There is no consensus on the definition of a compression fracture of the spine.[21] Developmental changes, degenerative disease, scoliosis, and kyphosis can cause vertebral deformities that can simulate fractures. Ferrar and colleagues[22] and Masharawi and colleagues[23] stated that short vertebral height without end plate fracture may be unrelated to osteoporosis and that quantitative morphometry alone

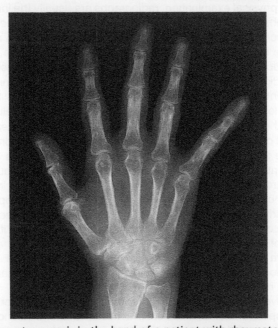

Fig. 4. Periarticular osteoporosis in the hand of a patient with rheumatoid arthritis.

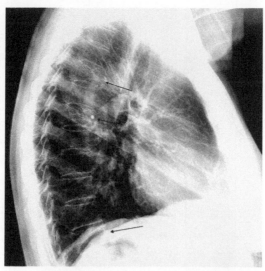

Fig. 5. Lateral view of a chest radiograph with compression fractures of the thoracic spine (*arrows*).

should not be used for assessment of vertebral fracture. Quantitative methods use morphometric measurements of heights of the end plates and areas of the vertebral bodies but are limited by difficulties in precisely determining the points for measurement.[24] The Genant classification of compression fractures is a semiquantitative method using both visual inspection and measurements.[25] The 3 types of vertebral deformity are anterior wedging with the anterior height decreased, crush with both the anterior and posterior heights decreased compared with adjacent vertebrae, and biconcave with the central vertebral height decreased compared with the anterior and posterior. A mild compression fracture is considered a 20% to 25% change, moderate 25% to 40%, and severe 40% and more. The Genant method uses both qualitative and quantitative assessment. Mild compression fractures may be difficult to differentiate from other vertebral deformities and are less reliable for determining osteoporosis. In children with osteoporosis, biconcavity is frequent because the normal intervertebral disk indents the osteoporotic bone (**Fig. 6**). In elderly patients, wedging and compression are more common because the disks may be degenerated and softer than the bone. The shape of the vertebral bodies varies from the thoracic to the lumbar spine. In the midthoracic spine, the anterior height of the vertebral bodies is less than the posterior height, giving an appearance of anterior wedging, whereas in the lower lumbar spine the height of the posterior vertebral bodies may be less than the anterior, giving the appearance of posterior wedging. Jiang and colleagues[26] compared an algorithm-based quantitative approach for determining compression fractures with qualitative and semiquantitive approaches and found that poor agreement among the methods arose mainly from difficulty in differentiating fracture from nonfracture deformity. Scoliosis may make it difficult to assess for vertebral fractures (**Fig. 7**). When the end plates of the vertebrae are not tangential to the x-ray beam (parallax), it may give the appearance of biconcavity. Schmorl nodes (disk herniation into the end plates) may be difficult to differentiate from end plate fractures. Large Schmorl nodes may be due to osteoporosis from weakening of the end plate, allowing disk protrusion through the end plate.

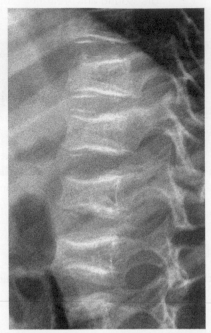

Fig. 6. Lumbar spine in a child with osteogenesis imperfecta; there is biconcavity of the vertebral bodies.

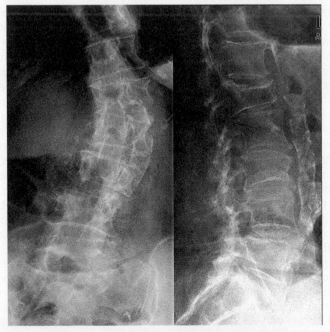

Fig. 7. AP and lateral of lumbar spine shows scoliosis and compression fracture of L1, L3 and L4 are difficult to evaluate because of parallax.

Routine CT and MRI are more specific than radiography in differentiating pathologic compression fractures due to neoplastic disease from osteoporotic compression fractures because they can detect bone destruction with lytic lesions and adjacent soft tissue mass. CT has better resolution than radiography for assessing end plate deformities and bone architecture. On MRI, acute compression fractures show decreased signal on T1 images and increased signal (bone marrow edema pattern) on T2 images or short tau inversion recovery (water-sensitive) images (**Fig. 8**). Both acute osteoporotic and neoplastic compression fractures show high signal on water-sensitive images. On T1 images, however, osteoporotic fractures usually show only partial replacement of bone marrow (**Fig. 9**A) whereas neoplastic fractures usually show complete replacement of the marrow in the vertebral body.[27] The high signal on the water-sensitive images usually reverts to normal within 1 to 3 months in an osteoporotic compression fracture, which helps determine the chronicity of the fracture (**Fig. 9**B).

Radionuclide bone scanning can be done using gamma cameras, with injection of technetium Tc 99m phosphate complexes, or using positron emission tomography scanners with injection of Fluorine-18. Both can be combined with simultaneous CT scanning for precise localization of the site of the abnormal increased uptake of the radionuclide. Whole-body scanning using these technologies may detect atraumatic fractures that may not be clinically suspected or that may not be visible on radiography. Increased uptake in compression fractures of the spine usually reverts to normal in approximately 6 months but can be present longer if there is continued collapse of the vertebral body or continued remodeling of bony deformity. Quantitative radionuclide scanning has been used in research studies to evaluate bone turnover.

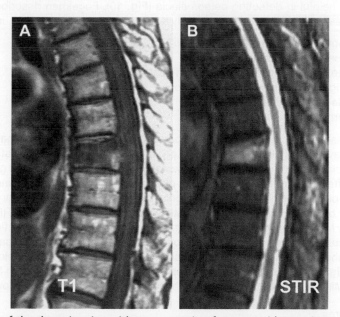

Fig. 8. MRI of the thoracic spine with a compression fracture, with anterior wedging of a thoracic vertebral body. The T1 (*A*) image shows decreased signal in the fractured vertebral body because of the marrow edema pattern. The remaining vertebral bodies have normal high signal on T1 from marrow fat. The short tau inversion recovery (STIR) (*B*) image shows bright signal in the compression fracture due to the marrow edema pattern, whereas the remaining normal vertebral bodies have low signal from the fat suppression sequence.

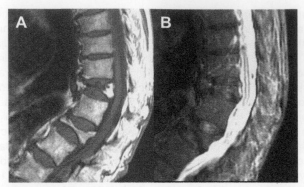

Fig. 9. MRI of spine with chronic osteoporotic compression fractures. (*A*) TI image shows some remaining increased signal, indicating that all of the marrow was not replaced. (*B*) T2 image does not show marrow edema pattern (increased signal), indicating the fractures are chronic.

Bisphosphonate therapy for osteoporosis decreases bone turnover and suppresses bone uptake of radionuclide.[28] Teriparatide therapy increases osteoblastic activity and increases uptake of radionuclide.[29] Osteomalacia, hyperparathyroidism, and renal osteodystrophy cause high bone turnover that may be seen as a high bone-to–soft tissue uptake ratio on bone scanning. Osteoporosis usually is not a high bone turnover disease and shows normal or low bone-to–soft tissue ratio.

Osteomalacia can cause low bone density and has to be differentiated from osteoporosis because the causes and the treatment are not the same. Radionuclide bone scanning is helpful in detecting osteomalacia (**Fig. 10**). Fogelman described "metabolic features" on bone scans that strongly suggest a metabolic disorder, including[30]

- High bone-to–soft tissue uptake ratio
- Increased uptake around the joints
- Multiple insufficiency fractures, often bilateral
- Beading of the costochondral junctions
- Multiple rib fractures in a row
- Tie sternum

Osteomalacia may cause generalized bone and joint pain and muscle weakness that clinically may be mistaken for inflammatory arthritis. Some cases of osteomalacia (osteomalacia tumor induced) are due to excessive production of fibroblast growth factor 23 by often benign tumors, known as phosphaturic mesenchymal tumors, which cause hypophosphatemia.[31] Less commonly, the tumors may be malignant.[32] These tumors may be occult, and imaging modalities, including routine CT and MRI scanning, whole-body MRI scanning, and positron emission tomography Fluorine-18 fluorodeoxyglucose scanning, and Indium-111 Octreotide scanning may help find these tumors.[33]

Bisphosphonate therapy for osteoporosis may be associated with atypical femoral fractures (**Fig. 11**).[34] According to the advisory committee of the American Society for Bone and Mineral Research, features of these fractures include[35] the following:

Major features
- Location in the subtrochanteric region or femoral shaft
- Transverse or short oblique orientation
- Minimal or no trauma
- A medial spike when the fracture is complete
- Absence of comminution

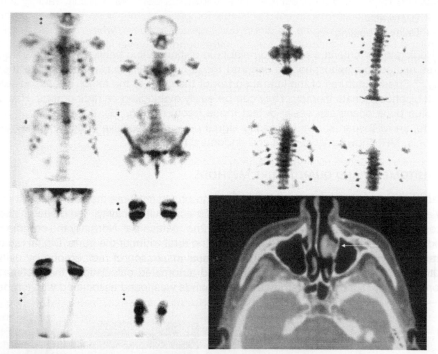

Fig. 10. Technetium Tc 99m bone scan shows features typical of osteomalacia, including multiple rib fractures in a row; beading of the costochondral junctions; insufficiency fractures of the femoral necks, metaphyseal regions of the distal femurs, and proximal and distal tibias; and high bone-to–soft tissue ratio. A mass (*arrow*) was found in the nasal cavity, on the CT scan (inset) which was a phosphaturic mesenchymal tumor. This is a frequent site of these tumors.

Minor features
- Association with cortical thickening
- Periosteal reaction of the lateral cortex
- Prodromal pain

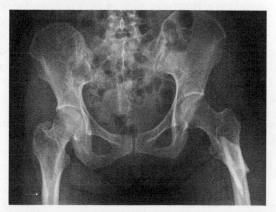

Fig. 11. Atypical femoral fracture of the left femur in a woman on bisphosphonate therapy. There is a stress fracture of the right femoral shaft (*arrow*) that later became a complete atypical femoral fracture.

- Bilaterality
- Delayed healing

Radiographic criteria were found reliable in distinguishing between complete fractures related to bisphosphonate use and those not related to bisphosphonate therapy.[36] Stress fractures of the lateral cortex of the shaft of the femur are associated with bisphosphonate therapy. They can be easily overlooked on radiographs. Radionuclide bone scans can easily detect these fractures (**Fig. 12**). If the fractures are acute, an MRI scan shows increased signal on water-sensitive images. If they are chronic, MRI shows only cortical and endosteal thickening.

DENSITOMETRY AND QUANTITATIVE METHODS

Radiogrammetry is a method that uses radiographs to measure the cortical thickness of a bone relative to its total width or width of the medullary cavity. The measurement most frequently used is the midportion of the 2nd metacarpal. Normally the combined width of the cortex is approximately 50% of the total width of the bone. Digital radiogrammetry has improved on the ordinary visual inspection of radiographs by using automated detection of the bone edges and automated calculations that estimate bone density. Digital radiogrammetry of the hands was found associated with lumbar

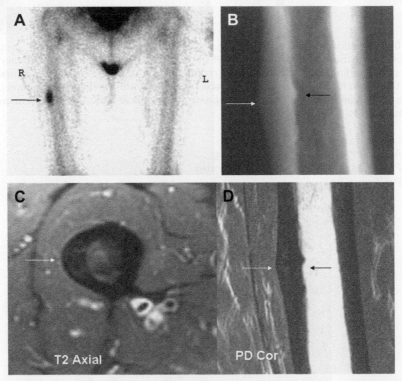

Fig. 12. (*A*) Focal increased uptake (*arrow*) in lateral femoral shaft on bone scan. (*B*) Cortical (*white arrow*) and endosteal thickening (*black arrow*) on radiograph. (*C*) MRI axial T2 with solid cortical thickening (*arrow*) and mild increased signal in the medullary cavity. (*D*) MRI coronal proton density with cortical (*white arrow*) and endosteal thickening (*black arrow*).

spine and total hip bone mineral density (BMD) by DXA in postmenopausal patients with rheumatoid arthritis.[37] Bone loss determined by digital radiogrammetry has been used to predict the onset of rheumatoid arthritis,[38] assess the activity and severity of inflammatory arthritis,[39,40] and assess treatment of bone loss.[41]

Quantitative evaluation of bone density on radiographs can be done by radiographic absorptiometry by obtaining plain digital radiographs, usually of the hands, along with an aluminum step wedge used as an internal reference, and computerized determination of absorption of the radiographs with linear regression analysis. Although postprocessing and acquisition settings can affect the results, Kinds and colleagues[42] found that reliable data may be obtained on bone density that may reduce the need for other methods.

The quantitative evaluation of bone density was revolutionized when instruments became available to measure bone density in the axial skeleton, mainly the lumbar spine and proximal femurs.[43] Before that, single-energy absorptiometers were able to measure density in the peripheral skeleton, such as the forearm or calcaneus, but not in the axial skeleton because of overlying soft tissue. Two energy sources enable subtraction of the soft tissues from the bone. Initially this was done with γ-rays from a radionuclide sources called dual-photon absorptiometry but later and more successfully with an x-ray source, DXA. Sites that are measured and that have normative databases are the lumbar spine (L1–L4), the proximal femur, the forearm, and the total body. The measurement is reported as BMD, which is the bone mineral content divided by the area. This is considered an areal density, using an estimation of the volume, and is reported in grams per square centimeter. Also reported are comparisons with normal databases for peak bone mass for young normal patients, ages 20 to 29 (T scores), and age-matched normal patients (z scores). In 1994, a WHO study group developed a diagnostic classification of osteopororosis based on the relationship between bone density, measured by DXA, and prevalence of fractures.

WHO Classification

The WHO classification should be used only for postmenopausal or transitional menopausal women and for men older than age 50. For others, z scores of lower than −2.0 should be reported as lower than the expected range and, if greater than −2.5, within the expected range.

- Normal: T score greater than −1.0 SD
- Osteopenia or low bone density: T score −1.0 to −2.5
- Osteoporosis: T score −2.5 or lower

Most clinicians follow the guidelines for DXA developed by the International Society for Clinical Densitometry (ISCD) that are available on its Web site (www.isgd.org) and that have been published.[44,45] In the spine, L1–L4 should be measured. Vertebrae should be excluded if their T score is more than 1 SD different from adjacent vertebrae or if there is structural change from degenerative disease or fracture (**Fig. 13**). At least 2 vertebrae should be included for diagnosis. In many patients, the spine cannot be used because of degenerative disease causing sclerosis or because of vertebral deformity. The femoral neck and total hip regions of interest should also be used for diagnosis (**Fig. 14**). The forearm one-third site of the nondominant arm can be used in some cases (**Fig. 15**). The one-third site of the forearm is 95% cortical bone (see **Fig. 15**). It can be useful in suspected hyperparathyroidism that has increased cortical bone loss and if the spine and proximal femurs cannot be measured. Other sites or the measurements from other modalities should not be used for WHO classification.

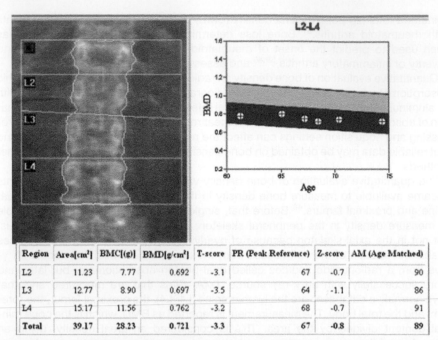

Region	Area[cm²]	BMC[(g)]	BMD[g/cm²]	T-score	PR (Peak Reference)	Z-score	AM (Age Matched)
L2	11.23	7.77	0.692	-3.1	67	-0.7	90
L3	12.77	8.90	0.697	-3.5	64	-1.1	86
L4	15.17	11.56	0.762	-3.2	68	-0.7	91
Total	39.17	28.23	0.721	-3.3	67	-0.8	89

Fig. 13. DXA scan of the lumbar spine of a 74-year-old woman. L1 was excluded because of a compression fracture. The T score for L2–L4 was −3.3, indicating a classification of osteoporosis. The graph compares the DXA bone densities over time.

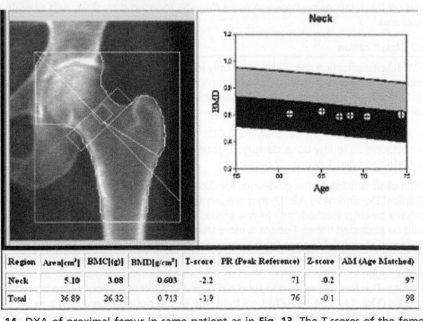

Region	Area[cm²]	BMC[(g)]	BMD[g/cm²]	T-score	PR (Peak Reference)	Z-score	AM (Age Matched)
Neck	5.10	3.08	0.603	-2.2	71	-0.2	97
Total	36.89	26.32	0.713	-1.9	76	-0.1	98

Fig. 14. DXA of proximal femur in same patient as in **Fig. 13**. The T scores of the femoral neck and total hip are not in the range of osteoporosis; however, for classification, the lowest T score of the scanned sites is used. Only the femoral neck and total hip regions of the proximal femur are used.

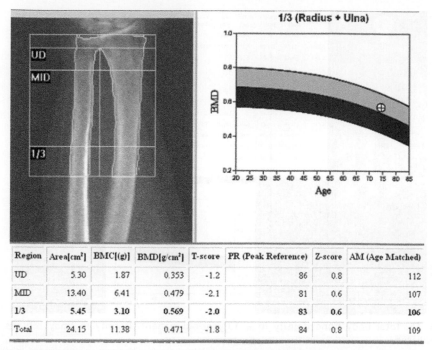

Region	Area[cm²]	BMC[(g)]	BMD[g/cm²]	T-score	PR (Peak Reference)	Z-score	AM (Age Matched)
UD	5.30	1.87	0.353	-1.2	86	0.8	112
MID	13.40	6.41	0.479	-2.1	81	0.6	107
1/3	5.45	3.10	0.569	-2.0	83	0.6	106
Total	24.15	11.38	0.471	-1.8	84	0.8	109

Fig. 15. DXA of forearm in the same patient as in **Figs. 13** and **14**. Only the one-third site is used.

Lateral scanning of the lumbar spine provides a region of interest that is predominantly cancellous bone, which has a higher bone turnover, but lateral scanning is seldom used in clinical practice and should not be used for WHO classification. For pediatric patients (under 19 years old), the lumbar spine and total body are measured (**Fig. 16**). DXA can be done at peripheral skeletal sites other than forearm, including the calcaneus and hand. Peripheral sites should not be used for monitoring therapy. DXA is recommended for women 65 and older, men 70 and older, postmenopausal women with risk factors for fracture, patients with fragility fractures, and patients with diseases associated with low bone density or who are on or going on medication associated with low bone density (such as glucocorticoids). Total-body DXA provides body composition analysis, giving percentage of body fat and lean muscle mass (**Fig. 17**). Evaluation of sarcopenia is becoming an important in studying and treating patients with osteoporosis.[46]

The ability to monitor bone loss or gain by DXA depends on the amount of change and the precision of the DXA measurements. The precision can be calculated by scanning 15 patients 3 times each or 30 patients twice and then calculating the precision in BMD or coefficient of variation. A spreadsheet and calculator for precision are available on the ISCD Web site. With a 95% confidence, the least significant change (LSC) is 2.77 × the precision. The ISCD guidelines state that the minimum precision for the lumbar spine should be 1.9% (LSC = 5.3%; femoral neck 2.5% [LSC = 6.9%]; total hip 1.8% [LSC = 5.0%]). Medicare and most insurance companies approve DXA every 2 years but may approve it more frequently in patients treated for rheumatic diseases with agents, such as corticosteroids, that commonly produce rapid bone loss. In many patients, the rate of change in bone density, before

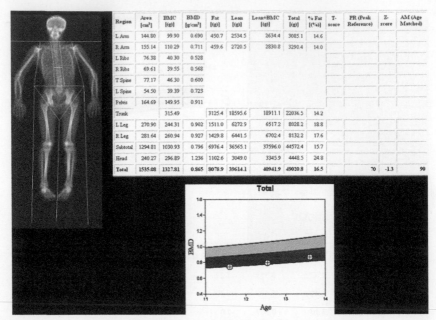

Region	Area [cm²]	BMC [(g)]	BMD [g/cm²]	Fat [(g)]	Lean [(g)]	Lean+BMC [(g)]	Total [(g)]	% Fat [(%)]	T-score	PR (Peak Reference)	Z-score	AM (Age Matched)
L Arm	144.80	99.90	0.690	450.7	2534.5	2634.4	3085.1	14.6				
R Arm	155.14	110.29	0.711	459.6	2720.5	2830.8	3290.4	14.0				
L Ribs	76.38	40.30	0.528									
R Ribs	69.61	39.55	0.568									
T Spine	77.17	46.30	0.600									
L Spine	54.50	39.39	0.723									
Pelvis	164.69	149.95	0.911									
Trunk		315.49		3125.4	18595.6	18911.1	22036.5	14.2				
L Leg	270.90	244.31	0.902	1511.0	6272.9	6517.2	8028.2	18.8				
R Leg	281.64	260.94	0.927	1429.8	6441.5	6702.4	8132.2	17.6				
Subtotal	1294.81	1030.93	0.796	6976.4	36565.1	37596.0	44572.4	15.7				
Head	240.27	296.89	1.236	1102.6	3049.0	3345.9	4448.5	24.8				
Total	1535.08	1327.81	0.865	8078.9	39614.1	40941.9	49020.8	16.5		70	-1.3	90

Fig. 16. Total body bone density in a 13-year-old patient. Density in body regions is calculated.

Measure	Scan Date	Age	Result	YN %ile	AM %ile	Change vs Baseline	Change vs Previous
Total Body % Fat	01/23/2013	13	16.5		5	-6.3	-1.7
	12/28/2011	12	18.2		7	-4.6	-4.6
	01/17/2011	11	22.8		27		

Measure	Scan Date	Age	Result	Change/Month vs Baseline	Change/Month vs Previous	Change vs Baseline	Change vs Previous
Total Fat Mass	01/23/2013	13	8079	43	84	1041	1085
	12/28/2011	12	6994	-4	-4	-44	-44
	01/17/2011	11	7038				

Measure	Scan Date	Age	Result	Change/Month vs Baseline	Change/Month vs Previous	Change vs Baseline	Change vs Previous
Total Lean+BMC Mass	01/23/2013	13	40942	706	742	17081	9538
	12/28/2011	12	31404	667	667	7544	7544
	01/17/2011	11	23861				

Measure	Scan Date	Age	Result	Change/Month vs Baseline	Change/Month vs Previous	Change vs Baseline	Change vs Previous
Total Mass	01/23/2013	13	49021	749	827	18123	10623
	12/28/2011	12	38398	664	664	7500	7500
	01/17/2011	11	30898				

Fig. 17. Body composition results from the same 13 y/o patient in **Fig. 16.** Total body percentage of fat, total fat mass, total lean plus bone mineral content mass, and total mass were measured.

and after bisphosphonate therapy, is not high enough to detect the results in 1 to 2 years or even more by measuring BMD. The use of biomarkers can supplement BMD in risk assessment and monitoring therapy.[47] Markers of bone resorption include the breakdown products of type I collagen, N-telopeptide and C-terminal peptide, which decrease within months after bisphosphonate therapy. Elevation of these markers indicates increased bone turnover. Markers of bone formation include bone-specific alkaline phosphatase, osteocalcin, and the carboxy and aminoterminal propeptides of type I procollagen, PICP and PINP.

BMD levels correlate with bone strength and fracture risk.[48,49] The rule of thumb is that for each 1 SD decrease in BMD the fracture risk approximately doubles. There are other factors, however, that are important in predicting fracture risk. Age is important because fractures are not common in younger patients with low bone density when compared with similar bone density in older patients. The fracture risk assessment tool (FRAX) was developed to predict the 10-year risk of major osteoporotic fractures and hip fractures.[50–52] Factors that are placed in the calculator are

- DXA measurement of femoral neck BMD
- Age
- Gender
- Height
- Weight
- Previous fracture
- Hip fracture in parent
- Smoking
- Glucocorticoid use
- Rheumatoid arthritis
- Secondary osteoporosis
- 3 or More units of alcohol consumption per day
- Country

FRAX is not used in patients who have been on pharmacologic therapy for osteoporosis because these drugs alter fracture risk. Treatment of osteoporosis can be based on the fracture risk calculated by FRAX rather than on BMD alone. A National Osteoporosis Foundation guideline suggests implementation of pharmacologic therapy if there is a 10-year risk of a major osteoporotic fracture of 20% or more and hip fracture of 3% or more.[53] This may alter initiation of osteoporosis therapy to older patients, who are at a higher fracture risk, as opposed to younger patients with low bone density, who have a lower fracture risk.

Vertebral fracture assessment by DXA may be combined with bone densitometry by DXA to detect vertebral fractures.[54–57] Fractures are often present in patients who are not classified as osteoporotic by BMD measurement alone.[56] In vertebral fracture assessment, a scan is done by a DXA machine that allows the x-ray beam to be parallel to the end plates, diminishing the problem of parallax. Anteroposterior and lateral scans can be obtained of the thoracic and lumbar spine (**Fig. 18**). The radiation dose is only a small fraction of the radiation dose of routine anteroposterior and lateral spine radiographs.[58] An attempt is made to analyze the vertebrae from T4 to L4; however, there is sometimes inadequate visualization of the upper thoracic spine. The resolution of the images is not as good as with routine radiography. Automated or manual morphometric measurements can be done but are often inaccurate. The Genant semiquantitative method is used with both visual and morphometric analysis. Most moderate and severe compression fractures can de accurately detected; however, mild fractures may be missed.[55]

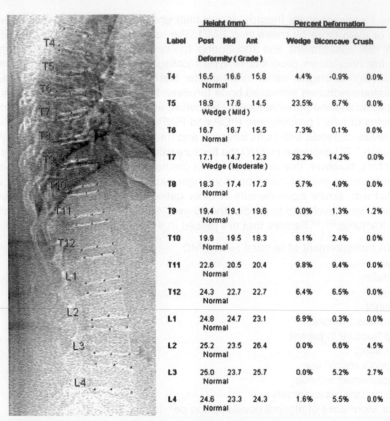

	Height (mm)			Percent Deformation		
Label	Post	Mid	Ant	Wedge	Biconcave	Crush
	Deformity (Grade)					
T4	16.5	16.6	15.8	4.4%	-0.9%	0.0%
	Normal					
T5	18.9	17.6	14.5	23.5%	6.7%	0.0%
	Wedge (Mild)					
T6	16.7	16.7	15.5	7.3%	0.1%	0.0%
	Normal					
T7	17.1	14.7	12.3	28.2%	14.2%	0.0%
	Wedge (Moderate)					
T8	18.3	17.4	17.3	5.7%	4.9%	0.0%
	Normal					
T9	19.4	19.1	19.6	0.0%	1.3%	1.2%
	Normal					
T10	19.9	19.5	18.3	8.1%	2.4%	0.0%
	Normal					
T11	22.6	20.5	20.4	9.8%	9.4%	0.0%
	Normal					
T12	24.3	22.7	22.7	6.4%	6.5%	0.0%
	Normal					
L1	24.8	24.7	23.1	6.9%	0.3%	0.0%
	Normal					
L2	25.2	23.5	26.4	0.0%	6.6%	4.5%
	Normal					
L3	25.0	23.7	25.7	0.0%	5.2%	2.7%
	Normal					
L4	24.6	23.3	24.3	1.6%	5.5%	0.0%
	Normal					

Fig. 18. Lateral scan done on the DXA machine for vertebral fracture assessment. The morphometric measurements show moderate wedging of T7 (*arrow*). On visual assessment, no end plate deformity is present. The patient had a normal bone density and no history of traumatic spine fracture. This is most likely a deformity due to degenerative or developmental change.

Quantitative CT (QCT) provides true volumetric measurements of bone density. It can separate cortical from cancellous bone. In the spine, it can avoid inclusion of peripheral osteophytes and vascular calcifications in the measurement of BMD. QCT can be done in the spine with single slices through the center of the vertebral bodies with comparison with a phantom of bone mineral equivalent (**Fig. 19**).[59–61] QCT can also be done without a phantom, with regions of interest in fat, muscle, and bone (**Fig. 20**). Volumetric CT allows 3-D imaging of the spine and proximal femur, at the cost of higher radiation doses than single slice. QCT can be done with ordinary CT scanners; however, software programs are needed for the calculations and normative databases. The center of the vertebral body, which is predominantly cancellous bone and has 8 times the bone turnover of cortical bone, is used and shows more rapid bone loss and greater response to therapy. QCT cannot be used for WHO classification. More patients with T scores below −2.5 are found with QCT than with DXA. QCT, however, does have a correlation with DXA.[62] The ISCD official position suggests that single-slice QCT be done from L1 to L3, and 3-D QCT from L1 to L2. Despite many of the advantages of QCT, DXA is the most frequent method used to measure bone density in clinical practice, with the most information available about BMD and fracture risk.

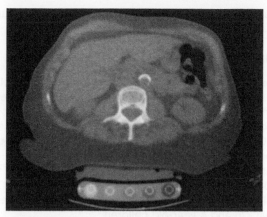

Fig. 19. QCT showing a single slice through the center of a lumbar vertebra with a bone mineral equivalent phantom beneath the patient.

Quantitative ultrasound densitometry (QUS) uses the measurement of the speed of sound through bone and the attenuation of sound in bone broadband ultrasound attenuation for evaluation of bone density. QUS densitometry machines are inexpensive and mobile, allowing them to be taken off-site. It is thought that bone architecture may also influence these 2 parameters, indicating mechanical properties of bone as well as BMD.[63] Measurements can be done in areas of the peripheral skeleton, including the calcaneus, radius, hand phalanges, and tibia, but cannot be used in the axial skeleton. QUS is not useful in monitoring therapy because the changes in measurements are too small. Correlation with bone density by DXA is only moderate.[64] QUS can be used to

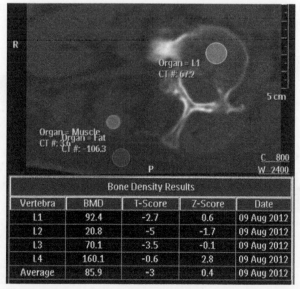

Bone Density Results				
Vertebra	BMD	T-Score	Z-Score	Date
L1	92.4	-2.7	0.6	09 Aug 2012
L2	20.8	-5	-1.7	09 Aug 2012
L3	70.1	-3.5	-0.1	09 Aug 2012
L4	160.1	-0.6	2.8	09 Aug 2012
Average	85.9	-3	0.4	09 Aug 2012

Fig. 20. QCT showing a single slice through one of the lumbar vertebral bodies scanned in a patient with scoliosis and degenerative disease of the spine. There is a marked variation in the density measurements of the vertebral bodies due to sclerosis from degenerative disease.

predict fracture risk and may be an independent predictor of fracture risk compared with BMD by DXA.[65]

ADVANCED IMAGING TECHNIQUES

New techniques have been developed for evaluating bone architecture.[4,66,67]

Peripheral QCT (pQCT) uses dedicated machines to scan peripheral sites, such as radius, tibia, and metacarpals. The XtremeCT (Scanco, Brütisellen, Switzerland) is a commercially available high-resolution pQCT scanner that can be used for the forearm and tibia. With pQCT, total, cortical, and cancellous BMD and area can be separately measured and bone architecture evaluated.[68–71] Cortical porosity can be seen. As opposed to DXA, It may be useful in following the effects of therapy.[72,73] pQCT is valuable in young children because it measures a volumetric density and is not affected by bone size. Bone size, not bone density, has been found to be correlated with weight and height in 3-year-old and 4-year-old children.[74,75]

MicroCT provides the best imaging resolution of bone architecture.[66] It requires biopsy bone specimens (**Fig. 21**). It can provide 3-D analysis of bone architecture.[76] Finite element analysis can be done, which provides models to assess bone strength and fracture risk of that bone.[77] In humans, biopsy specimens from the iliac crest are often used. Most experimental studies are done in laboratory animals.

Techniques have been developed for evaluation of bone density and trabecular bone structure by MRI of marrow susceptibility, which correlates with marrow fat, and bone volume fraction, which measures trabecular bone.[78,79] Routine sequences in MRI do not show signal in cortical bone. A new sequence, the ultrashort TE, allows water signal to be imaged in cortical bone and quantitation of MRI properties to be done, allowing MRI study of cortical bone.[80] The fat fraction in bone increases in osteoporosis. This can be measured by MRI spectroscopy. Finite element analysis can be used with MRI, CT, and DXA to evaluate bone architecture.[81–84] DXA can be used to assess femoral neck geometry, by determining hip axial length, femoral neck length, and femoral neck width, which are related to fracture risk.[85]

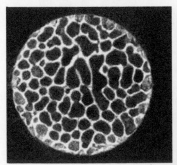

Vertebral core from a healthy adult ewe

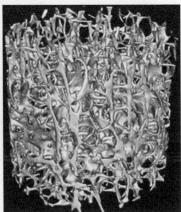

Iliac crest biopsy from an osteoporotic patient

Fig. 21. MicroCTs of a core specimen of the vertebral body of a healthy ewe (*left*) and of an osteoporotic human iliac crest biopsy left (at the Hospital for Special Surgery Musculoskeletal Repair and Regeneration Imaging Core).

REFERENCES

1. Bacchetta J, Boutroy S, Delmas PD, et al. New bone imaging techniques in children with chronic kidney disease. Arch Pediatr 2009;16(11):1482–90.
2. Wehrli FW, Saha PK, Gomberg BR, et al. Role of magnetic resonance for assessing structure and function of trabecular bone. Top Magn Reson Imaging 2002; 13(5):335–55.
3. Griffith JF, Genant HK. New advances in imaging osteoporosis and its complications. Endocrine 2012;42(1):39–51.
4. Link TM. Osteoporosis imaging: state of the art and advanced imaging. Radiology 2012;263(1):3–17.
5. Patsch JM, Burghardt AJ, Kazakia G, et al. Noninvasive imaging of bone microarchitecture. Ann N Y Acad Sci 2011;1240:77–87.
6. Guglielmi G, Muscarella S, Bazzocchi A. Integrated imaging approach to osteoporosis: state-of-the-art review and update. Radiographics 2011;31(5):1343–64.
7. Abdel Meguid MH, Hamad YH, Swilam RS, et al. Relation of interleukin-6 in rheumatoid arthritis patients to systemic bone loss and structural bone damage. Rheumatol Int 2013;33:697–703.
8. Hoes JN, Van der Goes MC, Jacobs JW, et al. Changes in macrophage inhibitory factor correlate with changes in bone mineral density in glucocorticoid-treated patients with rheumatoid arthritis. Rheumatology (Oxford) 2011;50(10):1921–4.
9. Geusens P, Lems WF. Osteoimmunology and osteoporosis. Arthritis Res Ther 2011;13(5):242.
10. Franck H, Braun J, Buttgereit F, et al, Kommission Osteologie der Deutschen Gesellschaft fur Rheumatologie. Bone densitometry in inflammatory rheumatic diseases: characteristics of the measurement site and disease-specific factors. Z Rheumatol 2009;68(10):845–50 [in German].
11. Njeh CF, Genant HK. Bone loss. Quantitative imaging techniques for assessing bone mass in rheumatoid arthritis. Arthritis Res 2000;2(6):446–50.
12. Yakemchuk V, Beaumont LF, Webber CE, et al. Vertebral fracture prevalence in a referral population of 750 Canadian men and women. Clin Radiol 2012;67(11): 1061–8.
13. Sbrocchi AM, Rauch F, Matzinger M, et al. Vertebral fractures despite normal spine bone mineral density in a boy with nephrotic syndrome. Pediatr Nephrol 2011;26(1):139–42.
14. Rauch F. Bone biopsy: indications and methods. Endocr Dev 2009;16:49–57.
15. Yamamoto N. Morphological analysis of bone dynamics and metabolic bone disease. Bone histomorphometry: the basic methods and role of bone research and clinical significance. Clin Calcium 2011;21(4):529–33 [in Japanese].
16. Ito A, Yajima A. Is bone biopsy necessary for the diagnosis of metabolic bone diseases? Necessity of bone biopsy. Clin Calcium 2011;21(9):1388–92.
17. Jorgetti V. Review article: bone biopsy in chronic kidney disease: patient level end-point or just another test? Nephrology (Carlton) 2009;14(4):404–7.
18. Pulkkinen P, Saarakkala S, Nieminen MT, et al. Standard radiography: untapped potential in the assessment of osteoporotic fracture risk. Eur Radiol 2012. [Epub ahead of print].
19. Haller J, Andre MP, Resnick D, et al. Detection of thoracolumbar vertebral body destruction with lateral spine radiography. Part I: investigation in cadavers. Invest Radiol 1990;25(5):517–22.
20. Majumdar SR, Kim N, Colman I, et al. Incidental vertebral fractures discovered with chest radiography in the emergency department: prevalence, recognition,

and osteoporosis management in a cohort of elderly patients. Arch Intern Med 2005;165(8):905–9.

21. Grados F, Fechtenbaum J, Flipon E, et al. Radiographic methods for evaluating osteoporotic vertebral fractures. Joint Bone Spine 2009;76(3):241–7.

22. Ferrar L, Jiang G, Armbrecht G, et al. Is short vertebral height always an osteoporotic fracture? The Osteoporosis and Ultrasound Study (OPUS). Bone 2007; 41(1):5–12.

23. Masharawi Y, Rothschild B, Peled N, et al. A simple radiological method for recognizing osteoporotic thoracic vertebral compression fractures and distinguishing them from Scheuermann disease. Spine (Phila Pa 1976) 2009;34(18): 1995–9.

24. Oei L, Rivadeneira F, Ly F, et al. Review of radiological scoring methods of osteoporotic vertebral fractures for clinical and research settings. Eur Radiol 2013; 23(2):476–86.

25. Genant HK, Wu CY, van Kuijk C, et al. Vertebral fracture assessment using a semiquantitative technique. J Bone Miner Res 1993;8(9):1137–48.

26. Jiang G, Eastell R, Barrington NA, et al. Comparison of methods for the visual identification of prevalent vertebral fracture in osteoporosis. Osteoporos Int 2004;15(11):887–96.

27. Baker LL, Goodman SB, Perkash I, et al. Benign versus pathologic compression fractures of vertebral bodies: assessment with conventional spin-echo, chemical-shift, and STIR MR imaging. Radiology 1990;174(2):495–502.

28. Frost ML, Siddique M, Blake GM, et al. Regional bone metabolism at the lumbar spine and hip following discontinuation of alendronate and risedronate treatment in postmenopausal women. Osteoporos Int 2012;23(8):2107–16.

29. Moore AE, Blake GM, Taylor KA, et al. Changes observed in radionuclide bone scans during and after teriparatide treatment for osteoporosis. Eur J Nucl Med Mol Imaging 2012;39(2):326–36.

30. Fogelman I, McKillop JH, Bessent RG, et al. The role of bone scanning in osteomalacia. J Nucl Med 1978;19(3):245–8.

31. Chong WH, Molinolo AA, Chen CC, et al. Tumor-induced osteomalacia. Endocr Relat Cancer 2011;18(3):R53–77.

32. Chiam P, Tan HC, Bee YM, et al. Oncogenic osteomalacia—hypophosphataemic spectrum from "benignancy" to "malignancy". Bone 2013;53(1):182–7.

33. Chong WH, Yavuz S, Patel SM, et al. The importance of whole body imaging in tumor-induced osteomalacia. J Clin Endocrinol Metab 2011;96(12):3599–600.

34. Gedmintas L, Solomon DH, Kim SC. Bisphosphonates and risk of subtrochanteric, femoral shaft, and atypical femur fracture: a systematic review and meta-analysis. J Bone Miner Res 2013. [Epub ahead of print].

35. Shane E, Burr D, Ebeling PR, et al. Atypical subtrochanteric and diaphyseal femoral fractures: report of a task force of the American Society for Bone and Mineral Research. J Bone Miner Res 2010;25(11):2267–94.

36. Rosenberg ZS, La Rocca Vieira R, Chan SS, et al. Bisphosphonate-related complete atypical subtrochanteric femoral fractures: diagnostic utility of radiography. AJR Am J Roentgenol 2011;197(4):954–60.

37. Desai SP, Gravallese EM, Shadick NA, et al. Hand bone mineral density is associated with both total hip and lumbar spine bone mineral density in postmenopausal women with RA. Rheumatology (Oxford) 2010;49(3):513–9.

38. de Rooy DP, Kalvesten J, Huizinga TW, et al. Loss of metacarpal bone density predicts RA development in recent-onset arthritis. Rheumatology (Oxford) 2012;51(6):1037–41.

39. Dirven L, Guler-Yuksel M, de Beus WM, et al. Changes in hand bone mineral density and the association with the level of disease activity in patients with rheumatoid arthritis: bone mineral density measurements in a multicenter randomized clinical trial. Arthritis Care Res (Hoboken) 2011;63(12):1691–9.

40. Pye SR, Adams JE, Ward KA, et al. Disease activity and severity in early inflammatory arthritis predict hand cortical bone loss. Rheumatology (Oxford) 2010; 49(10):1943–8.

41. Forsblad-d'Elia H, Carlsten H. Hormone replacement therapy in postmenopausal women with rheumatoid arthritis stabilises bone mineral density by digital x-ray radiogrammetry in a randomised controlled trial. Ann Rheum Dis 2011;70(6): 1167–8.

42. Kinds MB, Bartels LW, Marijnissen AC, et al. Feasibility of bone density evaluation using plain digital radiography. Osteoarthritis Cartilage 2011;19(11):1343–8.

43. Riggs BL, Khosla S, Melton LJ 3rd. Better tools for assessing osteoporosis. J Clin Invest 2012;122(12):4323–4.

44. Lewiecki EM, Gordon CM, Baim S, et al. International Society for Clinical Densitometry 2007 adult and pediatric official positions. Bone 2008;43(6): 1115–21.

45. Lewiecki EM, Gordon CM, Baim S, et al. Special report on the 2007 adult and pediatric Position Development Conferences of the International Society for Clinical Densitometry. Osteoporos Int 2008;19(10):1369–78.

46. Verschueren S, Gielen E, O'Neill TW, et al. Sarcopenia and its relationship with bone mineral density in middle-aged and elderly European men. Osteoporos Int 2013;24(1):87–98.

47. Garnero P. Biomarkers for osteoporosis management: utility in diagnosis, fracture risk prediction and therapy monitoring. Mol Diagn Ther 2008;12(3):157–70.

48. Haba Y, Lindner T, Fritsche A, et al. Relationship between mechanical properties and bone mineral density of human femoral bone retrieved from patients with osteoarthritis. Open Orthop J 2012;6:458–63.

49. Hsu JT, Chen YJ, Tsai MT, et al. Predicting cortical bone strength from DXA and dental cone-beam CT. PLoS One 2012;7(11):e50008.

50. Kanis JA, McCloskey EV, Johansson H, et al. Case finding for the management of osteoporosis with FRAX—assessment and intervention thresholds for the UK. Osteoporos Int 2008;19(10):1395–408.

51. Kanis JA, Oden A, Johansson H, et al. FRAX and its applications to clinical practice. Bone 2009;44(5):734–43.

52. Targownik LE, Bernstein CN, Nugent Z, et al. Inflammatory bowel disease and the risk of fracture after controlling for FRAX. J Bone Miner Res 2012. [Epub ahead of print].

53. Dawson-Hughes B, National Osteoporosis Foundation Guide Committee. A revised clinician's guide to the prevention and treatment of osteoporosis. J Clin Endocrinol Metab 2008;93(7):2463–5.

54. Guglielmi G, Diacinti D, van Kuijk C, et al. Vertebral morphometry: current methods and recent advances. Eur Radiol 2008;18(7):1484–96.

55. Fuerst T, Wu C, Genant HK, et al. Evaluation of vertebral fracture assessment by dual X-ray absorptiometry in a multicenter setting. Osteoporos Int 2009;20(7): 1199–205.

56. Jager PL, Slart RH, Webber CL, et al. Combined vertebral fracture assessment and bone mineral density measurement: a patient-friendly new tool with an important impact on the Canadian Risk Fracture Classification. Can Assoc Radiol J 2010;61(4):194–200.

57. Diacinti D, Guglielmi G. Vertebral morphometry. Radiol Clin North Am 2010;48(3): 561–75.
58. Vokes T, Bachman D, Baim S, et al. Vertebral fracture assessment: the 2005 ISCD Official Positions. J Clin Densitom 2006;9(1):37–46.
59. Cann CE, Genant HK. Precise measurement of vertebral mineral content using computed tomography. J Comput Assist Tomogr 1980;4(4):493–500.
60. Genant HK, Cann CE, Ettinger B, et al. The Classic: quantitative computed tomography of vertebral spongiosa: a sensitive method for detecting early bone loss after oophorectomy. 1982. Clin Orthop Relat Res 2006;443:14–8.
61. Engelke K, Adams JE, Armbrecht G, et al. Clinical use of quantitative computed tomography and peripheral quantitative computed tomography in the management of osteoporosis in adults: the 2007 ISCD Official Positions. J Clin Densitom 2008;11(1):123–62.
62. Cohen A, Lang TF, McMahon DJ, et al. Central QCT reveals lower volumetric BMD and stiffness in premenopausal women with idiopathic osteoporosis, regardless of fracture history. J Clin Endocrinol Metab 2012;97(11):4244–52.
63. Bouxsein ML, Radloff SE. Quantitative ultrasound of the calcaneus reflects the mechanical properties of calcaneal trabecular bone. J Bone Miner Res 1997; 12(5):839–46.
64. Grampp S, Genant HK, Mathur A, et al. Comparisons of noninvasive bone mineral measurements in assessing age-related loss, fracture discrimination, and diagnostic classification. J Bone Miner Res 1997;12(5):697–711.
65. Chan MY, Nguyen ND, Center JR, et al. Absolute fracture-risk prediction by a combination of calcaneal quantitative ultrasound and bone mineral density. Calcif Tissue Int 2012;90(2):128–36.
66. Genant HK, Engelke K, Prevrhal S. Advanced CT bone imaging in osteoporosis. Rheumatology (Oxford) 2008;47(Suppl 4):iv9–16.
67. Ito M. Recent progress in bone imaging for osteoporosis research. J Bone Miner Metab 2011;29(2):131–40.
68. Fouque-Aubert A, Boutroy S, Marotte H, et al. Assessment of hand bone loss in rheumatoid arthritis by high-resolution peripheral quantitative CT. Ann Rheum Dis 2010;69(9):1671–6.
69. Aeberli D, Eser P, Bonel H, et al. Reduced trabecular bone mineral density and cortical thickness accompanied by increased outer bone circumference in metacarpal bone of rheumatoid arthritis patients: a cross-sectional study. Arthritis Res Ther 2010;12(3):R119.
70. Morakis A, Tournis S, Papakitsou E, et al. Decreased tibial bone strength in postmenopausal women with aseptic loosening of cemented femoral implants measured by peripheral quantitative computed tomography (pQCT). J Long Term Eff Med Implants 2011;21(4):291–7.
71. Rubinacci A, Tresoldi D, Scalco E, et al. Comparative high-resolution pQCT analysis of femoral neck indicates different bone mass distribution in osteoporosis and osteoarthritis. Osteoporos Int 2012;23(7):1967–75.
72. Takada J, Iba K, Yamashita T. Diagnostic imaging of treatment in osteoporosis: SERM. Clin Calcium 2011;21(7):1047–55.
73. Tournis S, Samdanis V, Psarelis S, et al. Effect of rheumatoid arthritis on volumetric bone mineral density and bone geometry, assessed by peripheral quantitative computed tomography in postmenopausal women treated with bisphosphonates. J Rheumatol 2012;39(6):1215–20.
74. Binkley TL, Specker BL. pQCT measurement of bone parameters in young children: validation of technique. J Clin Densitom 2000;3(1):9–14.

75. Kalkwarf HJ, Laor T, Bean JA. Fracture risk in children with a forearm injury is associated with volumetric bone density and cortical area (by peripheral QCT) and areal bone density (by DXA). Osteoporos Int 2011;22(2):607–16.

76. Wang H, Ji B, Liu XS, et al. Analysis of microstructural and mechanical alterations of trabecular bone in a simulated three-dimensional remodeling process. J Biomech 2012;45(14):2417–25.

77. Evans SP, Parr WC, Clausen PD, et al. Finite element analysis of a micromechanical model of bone and a new 3D approach to validation. J Biomech 2012;45(15): 2702–5.

78. Lammentausta E, Hakulinen MA, Jurvelin JS, et al. Prediction of mechanical properties of trabecular bone using quantitative MRI. Phys Med Biol 2006;51(23): 6187–98.

79. Wehrli FW, Song HK, Saha PK, et al. Quantitative MRI for the assessment of bone structure and function. NMR Biomed 2006;19(7):731–64.

80. Du J, Bydder GM. Qualitative and quantitative ultrashort-TE MRI of cortical bone. NMR Biomed 2012. [Epub ahead of print].

81. Graeff C, Marin F, Petto H, et al. High resolution quantitative computed tomography-based assessment of trabecular microstructure and strength estimates by finite-element analysis of the spine, but not DXA, reflects vertebral fracture status in men with glucocorticoid-induced osteoporosis. Bone 2013;52(2): 568–77.

82. Danielson ME, Beck TJ, Karlamangla AS, et al. A comparison of DXA and CT based methods for estimating the strength of the femoral neck in postmenopausal women. Osteoporos Int 2012. [Epub ahead of print].

83. Naylor KE, McCloskey EV, Eastell R, et al. The use of DXA based finite element analysis of the proximal femur in a longitudinal study of hip fracture. J Bone Miner Res 2012. [Epub ahead of print].

84. Alberich-Bayarri A, Marti-Bonmati L, Angeles Perez M, et al. Assessment of 2D and 3D fractal dimension measurements of trabecular bone from high-spatial resolution magnetic resonance images at 3 T. Med Phys 2010;37(9):4930–7.

85. Dincel VE, Sengelen M, Sepici V, et al. The association of proximal femur geometry with hip fracture risk. Clin Anat 2008;21(6):575–80.

Tracking Rheumatic Disease Through Imaging

Carolyn M. Sofka, MD

KEYWORDS

- Radiographs • Nuclear imaging • Computed tomography • Ultrasonography
- Magnetic resonance imaging • Molecular imaging

KEY POINTS

- The use of imaging has rapidly evolved over the past 50 years, paralleling its increasing role in the diagnosis, monitoring, and follow-up of patients with rheumatic conditions.
- At present, radiographs are the mainstay of imaging, although magnetic resonance imaging and ultrasonography are routinely used for early diagnosis of disease, specifically for the identification of subclinical synovitis and erosions in rheumatoid arthritis.
- Computed tomography remains useful in evaluating the extent of involvement of inflammatory spondyloarthropathies that classically involve the axial skeleton and sacroiliac joints.
- Molecular imaging will likely play a key role in the future imaging of rheumatic conditions (specifically rheumatoid arthritis), with very specific and targeted tracers being used to identify early subclinical disease activity.

INTRODUCTION

Imaging has played an integral role in the diagnosis of rheumatologic conditions since the development of the radiograph.[1] Over the years, the role of imaging has changed from a purely diagnostic technique, often only obtained after symptoms have been present for some time, to that of an earlier diagnostic tool, with the intent to identify disease sooner, thus leading to earlier initiation of treatment with the ultimate goal of halting structural bone damage. In addition, providing an objective outcomes measure of various therapies, including specific targeted biological agents, has advanced the role of imaging to that of a key component in the diagnostic workup and clinical follow-up of patients with rheumatic diseases. More recently, molecular imaging has begun to play an innovative role in evaluating patients with arthritis, aiming to identify disease earlier and provide greater specificity. This review recounts the historical, current, and future involvement of radiology and imaging in the diagnosis, management, and follow-up of patients with various rheumatic conditions.

This work received Institutional Review Board approval.
Department of Radiology and Imaging, Hospital for Special Surgery, Weill Medical College of Cornell University, 535 East 70th Street, New York, NY 10021, USA
E-mail address: sofkac@hss.edu

Rheum Dis Clin N Am 39 (2013) 633–644
http://dx.doi.org/10.1016/j.rdc.2013.02.003
0889-857X/13/$ – see front matter © 2013 Elsevier Inc. All rights reserved.

RADIOGRAPHS AND NUCLEAR SCINTIGRAPHY

Conventional radiographs played the earliest role in the diagnosis of rheumatic conditions. Identification of erosions, joint-space narrowing, and distribution of disease were, and continue to be, invaluable to the rheumatologist in making a definitive diagnosis and, therefore, in instituting accurate and appropriate treatment (**Fig. 1**). Gradually the radiographic patterns of various arthritides were defined: the radiographic pattern of polyarthritis in reactive arthritis (formerly known as Reiter syndrome), for example, was elucidated in 1971.[2] In addition, specialized radiographic views have been developed throughout the years, increasing the diagnostic capabilities of radiographs and resulting in improved visualization of small joints, including those previously often obscured by other overlying osseous structures on routine frontal and lateral views (eg, the pisotriquetral joint view).[3]

Nuclear scintigraphy has also been used in the diagnosis of rheumatic conditions, primarily in the 1960s and 1970s (**Fig. 2**). The intravenous administration of strontium-85 (^{85}Sr) was one of the earliest radionuclide imaging methods used to identify bone marrow alterations in the setting of arthritis by localizing changes of osteoarthritis to either the medial or lateral compartments of the knee.[4] Furthermore, radioactive technetium (^{99m}Tc) was used to identify areas of active joint inflammation in a rheumatoid knee in comparison with a normal control.[5]

Nuclear scintigraphy has always been limited by its relatively low specificity; however, even early on, attempts were made to use radioactive tracers to better define bone marrow changes, specifically with respect to characterizing arthritis. In 1970 Muheim and Bohne[6] published their experience with using ^{85}Sr in 51 patients (52 knees) with supposed spontaneous osteonecrosis of the knee. Based on their

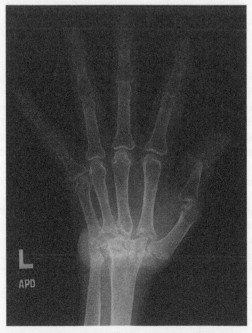

Fig. 1. Posteroanterior view of the left hand of a 65-year-old woman, demonstrating classic changes of rheumatoid arthritis with osteopenia, preferential proximal joint involvement in the carpus and carpometacarpal joints and erosions.

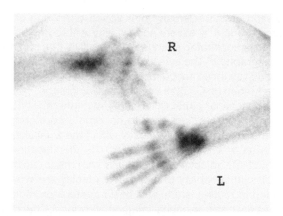

Fig. 2. Static images of the hands from a 3-phase bone scan in a 46-year-old woman with rheumatoid arthritis, demonstrating uptake throughout the carpus consistent with rheumatoid involvement.

conclusions, they suggested that nuclear scintimetry could potentially differentiate primary osteoarthritis from arthritis secondary to osteonecrosis.[6]

Radioactive tracers were used to further identify and characterize arthritis and their secondary complications throughout the early 1970s. Applications were expanded to include evaluation of the periarticular soft tissues, such as the identification of dissecting popliteal cysts, and soft-tissue changes in rheumatoid arthritis, such as tendinitis and bursitis.[7,8]

Nuclear scintigraphy was further used in the early 1970s to evaluate the axial skeleton, an area often visualized with some difficulty on conventional radiographs, such as the sacroiliac joints in ankylosing spondylitis.[9–11] Strontium-87m ([87m]Sr) demonstrated increased uptake in the sacroiliac joints in patients with active disease as demonstrated by both clinical presentation and laboratory values (erythrocyte sedimentation rate >40 mm/h).[9] Lentle and colleagues[10,11] not only identified the scintigraphic imaging findings throughout both the axial and appendicular skeletons in patients with ankylosing spondylitis, but also further emphasized the increased sensitivity of bone scintigraphy compared with conventional radiographs in diagnosing sacroiliac joint disease.

COMPUTED TOMOGRAPHY

As nuclear scintigraphy positioned itself to be an extremely sensitive diagnostic tool in the armamentarium of imaging for the diagnosis of rheumatic conditions in the 1970s, the relatively poor specificity necessitated a better imaging method to evaluate the regional anatomy in greater detail. The advent of computed tomography (CT) in the early 1980s allowed for a more detailed anatomic evaluation of articular surfaces, specifically those traditionally more difficult to evaluate with plain radiography, such as the sacroiliac joints and skull base.

Fam and colleagues[12] used CT to study 28 consecutive patients with low back pain and clinical findings suggestive of ankylosing spondylitis, and compared CT findings with routine radiographs of the sacroiliac joints. Each sacroiliac joint was evaluated using the standardized and previously validated New York criteria: grade 0 = normal; grade 1 = suspicious for erosions or sclerosis; grade 2 = mildly abnormal with definite erosions or sclerosis but without alteration in joint width; grade 3 = moderately abnormal with erosions, iliac and sacral sclerosis, joint space narrowing or widening, and/or partial ankylosis; and grade 4 = severe abnormality with complete ankylosis.[12,13] In 5 sacroiliac joints, CT demonstrated changes of sacroiliitis that had not been identified on conventional radiographs.[12] The investigators concluded that even mild sacroiliac joint abnormalities, such as those encountered with a relatively early disease presentation, were more clearly seen on CT than on routine radiographs.[12]

The tomographic multiplanar capabilities of CT, with the ability to perform sagittal and coronal reformatted images, lent itself to become a core element in imaging of patients with inflammatory disease, specifically within the axial skeleton (eg, spondyloarthropathies such as ankylosing spondylitis). The identification of erosions and malalignment at the C1-C2 articulation in patients with rheumatoid arthritis was now available through CT, with its ability to exquisitely identify the osseous structures in an area often clouded in routine lateral and flexion/extension radiographs, and with the added benefit of axial cross-sectional imaging allowing for the diagnosis of potential associated stenosis of the central canal (**Fig. 3**).[14]

Although CT has the relative limitation of ionizing radiation, it remains a key modality in the evaluation of patients with inflammatory conditions, especially the spondyloarthropathies whereby there is primarily involvement of the axial skeleton. Of significance, recent technological advances, such as iterative reconstruction techniques and imaging with fewer kilovolts, have resulted in diagnostic images with overall lower radiation dose to the patient, an important consideration in the pediatric and young adult population.

ULTRASONOGRAPHY

Ultrasonography began to be used to image clinical patients with suspected rheumatic disease in the late 1970s. Cooperberg and colleagues[15] assessed rheumatoid patients with knee synovitis with ultrasonography and compared findings with the

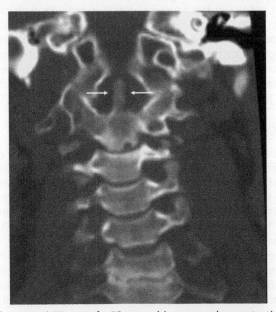

Fig. 3. Coronal reformatted CT scan of a 58-year-old woman, demonstrating erosive changes at the C1-C2 articulation eroding both the medial and lateral margins of the dens (*arrows*).

clinical presentation and conventional arthrography; this was the first description of the gray-scale appearance of synovial thickening and joint effusion in the knee. In 1988, ultrasonography was further expanded to evaluate tenosynovitis and synovitis in the hand in patients with rheumatoid arthritis, as well as to identify erosions.[16]

The 1990s then saw an exponential increase in the use of ultrasonography in the evaluation of rheumatic disease, primarily because of the availability and portability of ultrasound equipment, as well as the attractive feature of having no ionizing radiation. Improvements in transducer technology and software applications such as extended field of view and power Doppler resulted in increased diagnostic accuracy and validation of ultrasonography in the evaluation of inflammatory changes in rheumatic disease, and its adoption as a technology that aided the physician and the patient in therapeutic decision-making and assessing the response to treatment.[17]

In addition to the joint changes identifiable with ultrasonography such as synovitis and erosions, the sonographic appearance of normal and abnormal articular cartilage has been described. Grassi and colleagues[18] evaluated the distal femoral articular cartilage in normal subjects and those with osteoarthritis. Based on their examinations, the investigators defined the sonographic appearance of normal hyaline articular cartilage to be a homogeneous hypoechoic or anechoic band of tissue (given the high water content of normal cartilage) outlining the subchondral bone with a sharp superficial interface.[18] Abnormal, degenerated osteoarthritic cartilage, on the other hand, was identified by increased echogenicity of the articular cartilage (due to decreased water content), loss of the normal sharpness of the synovial-cartilage interface, loss of clarity of the cartilaginous layer, narrowing of the cartilage, and increased echogenicity of the posterior bone-cartilage interface.[18] Advanced applications such as this, capable of detailed evaluation of articular cartilage, have increased the diagnostic abilities of ultrasonography beyond that of simply identifying synovitis and erosions, and have positioned ultrasonography as a key modality in the imaging workup of patients with suspected rheumatic disorders.[19]

The use of ultrasonography has rapidly expanded beyond the identification and distribution of synovitis and erosions, primarily because of the development and application of power Doppler. Power Doppler imaging is an extremely sensitive detector of blood flow, being approximately 3 to 5 times more sensitive than conventional color Doppler.[20] It has the additional technical advantages of being angle independent and not affected by aliasing, thus allowing for technically easier scanning. Power Doppler has been validated in identifying areas of inflammation in both hip and knee synovitis, in combination with histopathology (**Fig. 4**).[21,22] Of importance, power

A   **B**

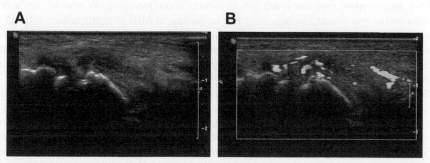

Fig. 4. Gray-scale (*A*) and power Doppler (*B*) images of the carpus demonstrate diffuse synovial thickening with visualization of marked active inflammatory changes when power Doppler is applied.

Doppler is very sensitive to states of slow blood flow, resulting in its ability to diagnose inflammation in small peripheral joints such as those involved in rheumatoid arthritis.[20] The tumor-like synovial proliferation in rheumatoid arthritis, in concert with the resultant increase in angiogenesis, is directly responsible for the increased blood flow seen with power Doppler.[23-25]

In addition to its utility in diagnosis, power Doppler ultrasonography is now used as a primary outcomes measure, monitoring response to therapy after injections or systemic treatment with disease-modifying antirheumatic drugs (DMARDs) (xenobiotic and biological agents).[26-28] Fiocco and colleagues[29] have shown that both gray-scale and power Doppler are reliable measures of disease activity in both rheumatoid and psoriatic knees. Furthermore, both power and spectral Doppler changes have been documented after treatment with systemic administration of tumor necrosis factor α blockers.[30-33] It has been shown that some patients who have been characterized by being in remission using the Disease Activity Score for 28 joints, the Clinical Disease Activity Index, or the Simplified Disease Activity Index actually have ultrasonographically defined active inflammation.[31,32] Thus there has been a recent call for the use of ultrasonography as a key component in defining "true" disease remission that has heretofore been based solely on clinical and laboratory test grounds.

MAGNETIC RESONANCE IMAGING

Cross-sectional imaging techniques further developed in the 1990s with the increased clinical use of magnetic resonance imaging (MRI). The increased soft-tissue resolution, combined with its tomographic imaging and the ability to identify areas of bone marrow edema pattern and, therefore, subclinical erosions has made MRI a key component in the imaging of patients with suspected rheumatic conditions. In 1990, Brown and colleagues[34] reported greater sensitivity of MRI in identifying inflammatory changes in the knee (synovitis, erosions, effusion, cartilage wear, and ligamentous/meniscal abnormality) compared with both clinical examination and routine radiography.

Use of MRI has rapidly expanded to include the evaluation of the small joints of the hand and wrist in patients with rheumatoid arthritis.[35-37] High-resolution surface coils and improved gradient platforms have resulted in the ability to identify and evaluate small joints of the hand and wrist, such as the metacarpophalangeal joints, for early changes of synovitis that have been shown to be the primary cause of bone damage in patients with rheumatoid arthritis (**Fig. 5**).[38]

MRI techniques can vary across facilities, thus resulting in some conflicting results within the literature regarding the accuracy of MRI in comparison with ultrasonography. MRI can be performed with or without an intravenous contrast agent (gadolinium [Gd-DTPA]), and the field strength and field of view can vary greatly (coned-down imaging of 1 or 2 joints, imaging of both hands at the same time, or even whole-body imaging).[39-41]

Some investigators advocate contrast-enhanced MRI in identifying early inflammatory changes. Jevtic and colleagues[42] evaluated 39 patients with a clinical diagnosis of ankylosing spondylitis with both contrast-enhanced Gd-DTPA MRI and radiographs, to evaluate for subtle changes at the discovertebral junctions. Contrast-enhanced MRI identified changes at the discovertebral junctions, suggesting early erosive changes compared with normal radiographic findings.[42] Furthermore, histologically it has been shown that there is a correlation of increased cellularity and resultant MRI enhancement in the setting of sacroiliitis in patients with spondyloarthopathies.[43]

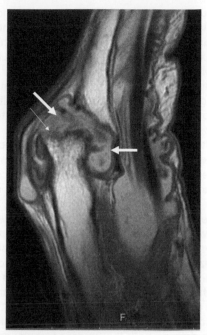

Fig. 5. Sagittal fast spin-echo proton-density weighted image of the left middle finger of a 49-year-old woman with rheumatoid arthritis demonstrates marked diffuse synovitis (*arrows*) with cortical bone loss primarily along the dorsal aspect of the head of the third metacarpal (*long thin arrow*) consistent with erosive disease.

Bollow and colleagues[43] found during a study of sacroiliac biopsies that T cells and macrophages are the most frequent types of cells infiltrating the sacroiliac joints in the early and active spondyloarthropathies, and that this degree of cellular infiltration correlated with the amount of gadolinium enhancement on MRI.

Similar to ultrasonography, the utility of MRI has expanded beyond the initial diagnosis to be an integral part of response to treatment and an objective outcomes measure. Quantitative improvement in a variety of disorders (rheumatoid arthritis, ankylosing spondylitis) after treatment with biological agents has been demonstrated with MRI. Braun and colleagues[44] reported significant reduction in spinal inflammation in patients with ankylosing spondylitis using MRI activity scores. Multiple studies have further demonstrated significant reduction in disease activity in patients with rheumatoid arthritis after treatment with DMARDs.[45–49]

MRI VERSUS ULTRASONOGRAPHY

There are often conflicting reports in the literature comparing and contrasting ultrasonography with MRI in the evaluation of patients with rheumatoid conditions, specifically peripheral small joint involvement, with regard to which is the "better" study.

Clearly both imaging modalities provide more diagnostic information than do radiographs alone, specifically with regard to soft-tissue changes of subclinical synovitis and erosions. It has been shown that both MRI and ultrasonography are much more sensitive than radiographs alone for the detection of erosions.[36,50] A direct comparison of the strengths and weaknesses of each modality by Rowbotham and Grainger[50] showed that neither modality emerged as the true "winner." Each has its own role in the evaluation of the rheumatoid patient. Certainly absolute and relative contraindications will limit the use of MRI in some patients (cochlear implants, pacemaker, or renal insufficiency in the setting of gadolinium administration), while the need to image deeper structures (the axial skeleton) will exclude the use of ultrasonography.

In comparison with MRI, ultrasonography is usually better tolerated by patients, especially those with claustrophobia; it is also usually less costly than MRI. Additional advantages of ultrasonography include the ability to image multiple joints in one sitting (without having to reposition the patient or the coil) and to perform diagnostic/therapeutic injections at the same sitting.

MRI produces exquisite anatomic images, perhaps more recognizable to those not frequently used to looking at ultrasonographic images. Moreover, with short-tau inversion recovery or frequency-selective fat-suppression techniques, MRI also has the ability to identify areas of bone marrow edema, thus diagnosing subclinical erosions.

Review of the literature often presents contradictory outcomes between ultrasonography and MRI for the evaluation of peripheral joint involvement in patients with rheumatoid arthritis; however, this is usually largely due to inconsistencies in study design and/or lack of standardization of MRI parameters or ultrasonographic techniques. A large meta-analysis performed in 2011 demonstrated that ultrasonography was more effective overall than radiographs for diagnosing erosions, and had efficacy comparable with that of MRI, with good reproducibility.[51]

The OMERACT (Outcome Measures in Rheumatology Clinical Trials) conferences have been paramount in defining both the ultrasonography and MRI criteria for joint synovitis and erosions, including defining quantitative or semiquantitative scoring systems that describe the degree of synovial/tenosynovial and erosive processes.[52] In further attempts to standardize imaging findings, the EULAR (European League Against Rheumatism)/OMERACT Ultrasound Task Force is in the process of developing a global OMERACT sonography scoring system (GLOSS) in rheumatoid arthritis, which examines small joints for synovitis using both gray-scale and power Doppler sonography scores.[53] Both imaging studies clearly play a role in the early diagnosis and follow-up of patients with rheumatoid disorders and should be viewed as complementary studies, with individualized studies tailored to the particular clinical question and patient characteristics. Recent initiatives from EULAR/OMERACT have further enhanced both methods of imaging by attempting to standardize findings and methods of reporting.[54–56]

THE FUTURE OF IMAGING IN RHEUMATOLOGY

The future of imaging in rheumatology will continue to build on the principle of early diagnosis and the use of standardized, sensitive, and reproducible outcomes measures for documenting the response to treatment. Newer MRI techniques including T1ρ and short echo-time imaging have potential clinical applications for the diagnosis of early cartilage damage in conditions such as osteoarthritis and rheumatoid arthritis.[57,58] More recently, the use of metabolic agents, such as ^{18}F-fluorodeoxyglucose positron emission tomography, and multi-pinhole single-photon emission CT has been applied to the evaluation of rheumatologic conditions, diagnosing subclinical disease activity with high sensitivity.[59–64] Lastly, metabolic agents have shown promise in the diagnosis, tracking, and monitoring of rheumatoid arthritis. Targeted imaging agents can be used to identify areas of active angiogenesis, and both nuclear and optical imaging methods of molecular imaging have been shown to be specific and sensitive for rheumatoid arthritis.[65]

SUMMARY

Imaging has played a key role in the diagnosis, monitoring, and determination of treatment outcomes in rheumatic conditions since the discovery of the radiograph. Various iterations in technology have resulted in better diagnostic tools, yielding earlier diagnosis of disease, thus resulting in earlier initiation of treatment, prevention of permanent bone damage and destruction, and, ultimately, functional limitation. Ultrasonography and MRI currently are the workhorses of peripheral joint evaluation in rheumatoid arthritis, being able to diagnose synovitis, erosions, and inflammation with greater sensitivity than conventional radiographs. Specific molecular imaging agents targeted to the variable disease pathology in rheumatoid arthritis hold promise for even more detailed, specific, and sensitive diagnosis of rheumatoid conditions, hopefully in its most early presentation and subclinical state, to aid in preventing the ultimate bone changes and patient discomfort that these diseases can produce.

REFERENCES

1. Huber N. Zur Verwerthung der Röntgen-Strahlen im Gebiete der inneren Medicin. Dtsch Med Wochenschr 1896;22(12):182–4 [in German].
2. Sholkoff SD, Glickman MG, Steinbach HL. The radiographic pattern of polyarthritis in Reiter's syndrome. Arthritis Rheum 1971;14(4):551–5.
3. Gardner-Thorpe D, Giddins GE. A reliable technique for radiographic imaging of the pisotriquetral joint. J Hand Surg Br 1999;24(2):252.
4. Bauer GC, Smith EM. ^{85}Sr scintimetry in osteoarthritis of the knee. J Nucl Med 1969;10(3):109–16.
5. Dick WC, Neufeld RR, Prentice AG, et al. Measurement of joint inflammation. A radioisotopic method. Ann Rheum Dis 1970;29(2):135–7.
6. Muheim G, Bohne WH. Prognosis in spontaneous osteonecrosis of the knee. Investigation by radionuclide scintimetry and radiography. J Bone Joint Surg Br 1970;52(4):605–12.
7. Levin MH, Nordyke RA, Ball JJ. Demonstration of dissecting popliteal cysts by joint scans after intra-articular isotope injections. Arthritis Rheum 1971;14(5):591–8.
8. Weissberg DL, Resnick D, Taylor A, et al. Rheumatoid arthritis and its variants: analysis of scintiphotographic, radiographic, and clinical examinations. AJR Am J Roentgenol 1978;131(4):665–73.
9. Van Laere M, Veys EM, Mielants H. Strontium 87m scanning of the sacroiliac joints in ankylosing spondylitis. Ann Rheum Dis 1972;31(3):201–6.
10. Lentle BC, Russell AS, Percy JS, et al. Scintigraphic findings in ankylosing spondylitis. J Nucl Med 1977;18(6):524–8.
11. Lentle BC, Russell AS, Percy JS, et al. The scintigraphic investigation of sacroiliac disease. J Nucl Med 1977;18(6):529–33.
12. Fam AG, Rubenstein JD, Chin-Sang H, et al. Computed tomography in the diagnosis of early ankylosing spondylitis. Arthritis Rheum 1985;28(8):930–7.
13. Bennet H, Wood PH. Population studies of the rheumatic diseases: Proceeding of the Third International Symposium, New York, June 1966. Amsterdam (Netherlands): Excerpta Medica; 1968. p. 456–7.
14. Lipson SJ. Cervical myelopathy and posterior atlanto-axial subluxation in patients with rheumatoid arthritis. J Bone Joint Surg Am 1985;67(4):593–7.
15. Cooperberg P, Tsang I, Truelove L, et al. Gray scale ultrasound in the evaluation of rheumatoid arthritis of the knee. Radiology 1978;126:759–63.
16. De Flaviis L, Scaglione P, Nessi R, et al. Ultrasonography of the hand in rheumatoid arthritis. Acta Radiol 1988;29:457–60.

17. Lund PJ, Heikal A, Maricic MJ, et al. Ultrasonographic imaging of the hand and wrist in rheumatoid arthritis. Skeletal Radiol 1995;24(8):591–6.

18. Grassi W, Lamanna G, Farina A, et al. Sonographic imaging of normal and osteoarthritic cartilage. Semin Arthritis Rheum 1999;28(6):398–403.

19. Kazam JK, Nazarian LN, Miller TT, et al. Sonographic evaluation of femoral trochlear cartilage in patients with knee pain. J Ultrasound Med 2011;30(6): 797–802.

20. Newman JS, Adler RS, Bude RO, et al. Detection of soft-tissue hyperemia: value of power Doppler sonography. AJR Am J Roentgenol 1994;163(2):385–9.

21. Walther M, Harms H, Krenn V, et al. Synovial tissue of the hip at power Doppler US: correlation between vascularity and power Doppler US signal. Radiology 2002;225(1):225–31.

22. Walther M, Harms H, Krenn V, et al. Correlation of power Doppler sonography with vascularity of the synovial tissue of the knee joint in patients with osteoarthritis and rheumatoid arthritis. Arthritis Rheum 2001;44(2):331–8.

23. Strunk J, Lange U. Three-dimensional power Doppler sonographic visualization of synovial angiogenesis in rheumatoid arthritis. J Rheumatol 2004;31(5):1004–6.

24. Schueller-Weidekamm C, Krestan C, Schueller G, et al. Power Doppler sonography and pulse-inversion harmonic imaging in evaluation of rheumatoid arthritis synovitis. AJR Am J Roentgenol 2007;188(2):504–8.

25. Freeston JE, Wakefield RJ, Conaghan PG, et al. A diagnostic algorithm for persistence of very early inflammatory arthritis: the utility of power Doppler ultrasound when added to conventional assessment tools [Erratum in Ann Rheum Dis 2011;70(8):1519]. Ann Rheum Dis 2010;69(2):417–9.

26. Naredo E, Collado P, Cruz A, et al. Longitudinal power Doppler ultrasonographic assessment of joint inflammatory activity in early rheumatoid arthritis: predictive value in disease activity and radiologic progression. Arthritis Rheum 2007; 57(1):116–24.

27. Salaffi F, Carotti M, Manganelli P, et al. Contrast-enhanced power Doppler sonography of knee synovitis in rheumatoid arthritis: assessment of therapeutic response. Clin Rheumatol 2004;23(4):285–90.

28. Filippucci E, Farina A, Carotti M, et al. Grey scale and power Doppler sonographic changes induced by intra-articular steroid injection treatment. Ann Rheum Dis 2004;63(6):740–3.

29. Fiocco U, Ferro F, Vezzù M, et al. Rheumatoid and psoriatic knee synovitis: clinical, grey scale, and power Doppler ultrasound assessment of the response to etanercept. Ann Rheum Dis 2005;64(6):899–905.

30. Takahashi A, Sato A, Yamadera Y, et al. Doppler sonographic evaluation of effect of treatment with infliximab (Remicade) for rheumatoid arthritis. Mod Rheumatol 2005;15(1):37–40.

31. Ribbens C, André B, Marcelis S, et al. Rheumatoid hand joint synovitis: grayscale and power Doppler US quantifications following anti-tumor necrosis factor-alpha treatment: pilot study. Radiology 2003;229(2):562–9.

32. Filippucci E, Iagnocco A, Salaffi F, et al. Power Doppler sonography monitoring of synovial perfusion at the wrist joints in patients with rheumatoid arthritis treated with adalimumab. Ann Rheum Dis 2006;65(11):1433–7.

33. Terslev L, Torp-Pedersen S, Qvistgaard E, et al. Estimation of inflammation by Doppler ultrasound: quantitative changes after intra-articular treatment in rheumatoid arthritis. Ann Rheum Dis 2003;62(11):1049–53.

34. Brown DG, Edwards NL, Greer JM, et al. Magnetic resonance imaging in patients with inflammatory arthritis of the knee. Clin Rheumatol 1990;9(1):73–83.

35. Fry ME, Jacoby RK, Hutton CW, et al. High-resolution magnetic resonance imaging of the interphalangeal joints of the hand. Skeletal Radiol 1991;20(4):273–7.

36. Poleksic L, Zdravkovic D, Jablanovic D, et al. Magnetic resonance imaging of bone destruction in rheumatoid arthritis: comparison with radiography. Skeletal Radiol 1993;22(8):577–80.

37. McQueen FM, Stewart N, Crabbe J, et al. Magnetic resonance imaging of the wrist in early rheumatoid arthritis reveals progression of erosions despite clinical improvement. Ann Rheum Dis 1999;58(3):156–63.

38. Conaghan PG, O'Connor P, McGonagle D, et al. Elucidation of the relationship between synovitis and bone damage: a randomized magnetic resonance imaging study of individual joints in patients with early rheumatoid arthritis. Arthritis Rheum 2003;48(1):64–71.

39. Hodgson RJ, O'Connor PJ, Ridgway JP. Optimizing MRI for imaging peripheral arthritis. Semin Musculoskelet Radiol 2012;16(5):367–76.

40. Weckbach S. Whole-body MRI for inflammatory arthritis and other multifocal rheumatoid diseases. Semin Musculoskelet Radiol 2012;16(5):377–88.

41. Althoff CE, Appel H, Rudwaleit M, et al. Whole-body MRI as a new screening tool for detecting axial and peripheral manifestations of spondyloarthritis. Ann Rheum Dis 2007;66(7):983–5.

42. Jevtic V, Kos-Golja M, Rozman B, et al. Marginal erosive discovertebral "Romanus" lesions in ankylosing spondylitis demonstrated by contrast enhanced Gd-DTPA magnetic resonance imaging. Skeletal Radiol 2000;29(1):27–33.

43. Bollow M, Fischer T, Reisshauer H, et al. Quantitative analyses of sacroiliac biopsies in spondyloarthropathies: T cells and macrophages predominate in early and active sacroiliitis—cellularity correlates with the degree of enhancement detected by magnetic resonance imaging. Ann Rheum Dis 2000;59(2):135–40.

44. Braun J, Baraliakos X, Golder W, et al. Magnetic resonance imaging examinations of the spine in patients with ankylosing spondylitis, before and after successful therapy with infliximab: evaluation of a new scoring system. Arthritis Rheum 2003;48(4):1126–36.

45. Lisbona MP, Maymó J, Perich J, et al. Rapid reduction in tenosynovitis of the wrist and fingers evaluated by MRI in patients with rheumatoid arthritis after treatment with etanercept. Ann Rheum Dis 2010;69(6):1117–22.

46. Østergaard M, Duer A, Nielsen H, et al. Magnetic resonance imaging for accelerated assessment of drug effect and prediction of subsequent radiographic progression in rheumatoid arthritis: a study of patients receiving combined anakinra and methotrexate treatment. Ann Rheum Dis 2005;64(10):1503–6.

47. Argyropoulou MI, Glatzouni A, Voulgari PV, et al. Magnetic resonance imaging quantification of hand synovitis in patients with rheumatoid arthritis treated with infliximab. Joint Bone Spine 2005;72(6):557–61.

48. Pedersen SJ, Sørensen IJ, Lambert RG, et al. Radiographic progression is associated with resolution of systemic inflammation in patients with axial spondyloarthritis treated with tumor necrosis factor α inhibitors: a study of radiographic progression, inflammation on magnetic resonance imaging, and circulating biomarkers of inflammation, angiogenesis, and cartilage and bone turnover. Arthritis Rheum 2011;63(12):3789–800.

49. Østergaard M, Emery P, Conaghan PG, et al. Significant improvement in synovitis, osteitis, and bone erosion following golimumab and methotrexate combination therapy as compared with methotrexate alone: a magnetic resonance imaging study of 318 methotrexate-naive rheumatoid arthritis patients. Arthritis Rheum 2011;63(12):3712–22.

50. Rowbotham EL, Grainger AJ. Rheumatoid arthritis: ultrasound versus MRI. AJR Am J Roentgenol 2011;197(3):541–6.
51. Baillet A, Gaujoux-Viala C, Mouterde G, et al. Comparison of the efficacy of sonography, magnetic resonance imaging and conventional radiography for the detection of bone erosions in rheumatoid arthritis patients: a systematic review and meta-analysis. Rheumatology (Oxford) 2011;50(6):1137–47.
52. Ohrndorf S, Backhaus M. Advances in sonographic scoring of rheumatoid arthritis. Ann Rheum Dis 2012. [Epub ahead of print].
53. D'Agostino MA, Said-Nahal R, Hacquard-Bouder C, et al. Assessment of peripheral enthesitis in the spondyloarthropathies by ultrasonography combined with power Doppler: a cross-sectional study. Arthritis Rheum 2003;48(2):523–33.
54. Bird P, Conaghan P, Ejbjerg B, et al. The development of the EULAR-OMERACT rheumatoid arthritis MRI reference image atlas. Ann Rheum Dis 2005;64(Suppl 1):i8–10.
55. Conaghan P, D'Agostino MA, Ravaud P, et al. EULAR report on the use of ultrasonography in painful knee osteoarthritis. Part 2: exploring decision rules for clinical utility. Ann Rheum Dis 2005;64(12):1710–4.
56. Østergaard M, McQueen FM, Bird P, et al, OMERACT 7 Special Interest Group. Magnetic resonance imaging in rheumatoid arthritis advances and research priorities. J Rheumatol 2005;32(12):2462–4.
57. Tsushima H, Okazaki K, Takayama Y, et al. Evaluation of cartilage degradation in arthritis using T1ρ magnetic resonance imaging mapping. Rheumatol Int 2012; 32(9):2867–75.
58. Insko EK, Reddy R, Leigh JS. High resolution, short echo time sodium imaging of articular cartilage. J Magn Reson Imaging 1997;7(6):1056–9.
59. Beckers C, Ribbens C, André B, et al. Assessment of disease activity in rheumatoid arthritis with (18)F-FDG PET. J Nucl Med 2004;45(6):956–64.
60. Seldin DW, Habib I, Soudry G. Axillary lymph node visualization on F-18 FDG PET body scans in patients with rheumatoid arthritis. Clin Nucl Med 2007;32(7):524–6.
61. Chaudhari AJ, Bowen SL, Burkett GW, et al. High-resolution (18)F-FDG PET with MRI for monitoring response to treatment in rheumatoid arthritis. Eur J Nucl Med Mol Imaging 2010;37(5):1047.
62. dos Anjos DA, do Vale GF, Campos Cde M, et al. Extra-articular inflammatory sites detected by F-18 FDG PET/CT in a patient with rheumatoid arthritis. Clin Nucl Med 2010;35(7):540–1.
63. Ostendorf B, Scherer A, Wirrwar A, et al. High-resolution multipinhole single-photon-emission computed tomography in experimental and human arthritis. Arthritis Rheum 2006;54(4):1096–104.
64. Elzinga EH, van der Laken CJ, Comans EF, et al. ^{18}F-FDG PET as a tool to predict the clinical outcome of infliximab treatment of rheumatoid arthritis: an explorative study. J Nucl Med 2011;52(1):77–80.
65. Wunder A, Straub RH, Gay S, et al. Molecular imaging: novel tools in visualizing rheumatoid arthritis. Rheumatology (Oxford) 2005;44(11):1341–9.

Imaging of Spondyloarthropathies

Mai Mattar, MD[a,b,*], David Salonen, MD[c],
Robert D. Inman, MD[d,e,f]

KEYWORDS

- Axial spondyloarthropathy (SpA) • Anatomy • Imaging modalities • Approach
- Differential considerations

KEY POINTS

- Plain radiography is the initial and standard method of investigation in axial SpAs. Careful evaluation of the radiographs through developing a systematic approach is indispensible in reaching the correct diagnosis.
- Cross-sectional imaging, in particular magnetic resonance imaging, has been increasingly used in evaluating SpAs in particular during the early phases of the disease or when radiographic findings are equivocal.
- Different types of SpAs demonstrate different imaging characteristics that are important to identify to reach the correct diagnosis.

INTRODUCTION

Spondyloarthropathies (SpA) refer to a group of disorders that primarily affect the synovial joints of the axial and appendicular skeleton of variable predilections.

SpA include the group's prototype ankylosing spondylitis (AS) as well as psoriatic arthritis, reactive spondyloarthropathy (previously called Reiter syndrome), and enteropathic spondylitis (or spondylitis of inflammatory bowel disease). This group shares spine and sacroiliac joint involvement with variable involvement of the peripheral

[a] Joint Department of Medical Imaging, Mount Sinai Hospital, Women's College Hospital, University Health Network, Toronto, Ontario, Canada; [b] Department of Medical Imaging, Toronto Western Hospital, 399 Bathurst Street, Fell Pavilion, 3rd Floor, Toronto, Ontario M5T 2S8, Canada; [c] Musculoskeletal Imaging, Department of Medical Imaging, Mount Sinai Hospital, University of Toronto, University Health Network, 600 University Avenue, Toronto, Ontario M5G 1X, Canada; [d] Medicine, University of Toronto, Toronto, Ontario, Canada; [e] Immunology, University of Toronto, Toronto, Ontario, Canada; [f] Research Medicine, Toronto Western Hospital, University Health Network, 1E-423, 399 Bathurst Street, Toronto, Ontario M5T 2S8, Canada
* Corresponding author. Department of Medical Imaging, Toronto Western Hospital, 399 Bathurst Street, Fell Pavilion, 3rd Floor, Toronto, Ontario M5T 2S8, Canada.
E-mail address: maimattar79@gmail.com

Rheum Dis Clin N Am 39 (2013) 645–667
http://dx.doi.org/10.1016/j.rdc.2013.02.005
0889-857X/13/$ – see front matter
rheumatic.theclinics.com

joints. They are commonly associated with the human leukocyte antigen B27 (HLA-B27) that explains their familial preponderance[1] and also correlates with the severity of the disease.[2]

Amongst other chronic inflammatory diseases, the prototype of the seropositive group is rheumatoid arthritis (RA), which affects primarily the peripheral joints with minor arthritis involvement of the spine.

In this article, the focus is on the pattern of spinal involvement in the axial skeleton, initially speaking about the relevant anatomy of the spine and sacroiliac joints. Then described are the imaging modalities most commonly used today, in addition to the standard imaging protocols for diagnosing and monitoring disease progression.

In the second part, an approach is formulated to evaluate the spine in inflammatory SpAs and the imaging patterns of specific disease entities are outlined, with a brief description of other pathologic processes that may affect the spine and sacroiliac joints and may mimic spondyloarthropathies.

OVERVIEW OF SPINAL ANATOMY

- There are 33 vertebrae (7 cervical, 12 thoracic, 5 lumbar, 5 sacral, and 4 coccygeal vertebrae). The number can vary from 32 to 35.
- The vertebra is usually divided into the body (the anterior bone mass) and the posterior elements or the neural arch, which consists of 2 pedicles and laminae, the spinous, transverse, and articular processes. The vertebral body morphology is slightly different in each segment of the spine.[3]
- The articular surfaces consist of the following:
  o The facet joints: zygoapophyseal and synovial joints formed by the superior and inferior facets. They tend to be involved in certain types of SpAs.
  o The intervertebral disc: acts to absorb and alleviate axial forces through the spine. It is composed of the 3 following distinct parts:
    ▪ The vertebral endplate: the hyaline cartilage that covers the superior and inferior surfaces of the vertebral bodies.
    ▪ The nucleus pulposus: the central, fluid-filled component of the disc. Water constitutes 85% to 90% of the nucleus, and collagen and proteoglycans account for most of the macromolecular constituents. The nucleus appears bright on fluid-sensitive magnetic resonance imaging (MRI) sequences.
    ▪ The annulus fibrosis: the outer, capsular component of the disc. Its central fibers blend with the nucleus and help to keep it in place. Its peripheral, ring-like fibers attach to the superior and inferior aspects of the vertebral body through Sharpey fibers and also attach to the anterior and posterior longitudinal ligaments.[4]
  o Ligaments:
    ▪ Anterior longitudinal ligament (ALL): a thick ligament that runs across the anterior aspect of the vertebral column from the skull to the sacrum.
    ▪ Posterior longitudinal ligament: A ligament that runs along the dorsum of the vertebrae from the skull to sacrum.
    ▪ Craniocervical and interspinous ligaments.

The normal ligaments appear as low signal intensity structures on all MRI sequences (**Fig. 1**).

For the purpose of this article, the anatomic description is limited to the osseous and articular structures.

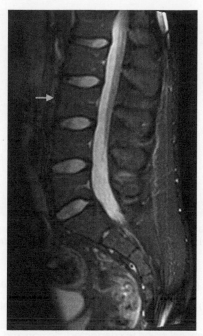

Fig. 1. Sagittal T2 fat-saturated image of the lumbar spine demonstrating normal vertebral body morphology, with low signal intensity seen in all the ligaments including the ALL (*arrow*) and the interspinous ligaments. Note the high T2 signal within the intervertebral disc reflecting its high water content.

OVERVIEW OF SACROILIAC JOINT ANATOMY

The sacroiliac joint (SIJ) is a complex S-shaped articulation between the iliac and sacral bones. It acts as a weight-bearing joint and demonstrates very limited gliding and rotation. It is normally divided into anterior and posterior components:

- Anterior component: referred to as the synovial joint, although only the inferior one-third and the anterior-most aspect of the superior component are truly synovial (**Fig. 2**A). The cartilage overlying the iliac aspect of the joint is thinner than the sacral aspect (2 and 3–5 mm, respectively); therefore, the changes of inflammatory arthropathies are observed on the iliac side first.
- Posterior component: a syndesmotic joint between the sacral and iliac tuberosities, traversed by strong interosseous sacroiliac ligaments that help maintain the alignment and transfer forces through the articular components (see **Fig. 2**B).
- Several ligaments run between the lower lumbar spine, iliac bone, and sacrum anteriorly and posteriorly, all of which contribute to joint stability.[5]

IMAGING EVALUATION OF AXIAL SPA
Plain Radiography

Plain (or conventional) radiography is the mainstream of SpA imaging. It is the first line of imaging evaluation due to its relative inexpensiveness, accessibility, and usefulness in monitoring disease progression. Imaging currently plays an important role in research defining the different classes of medications that may affect disease progression, in particular, new bone formation.[6]

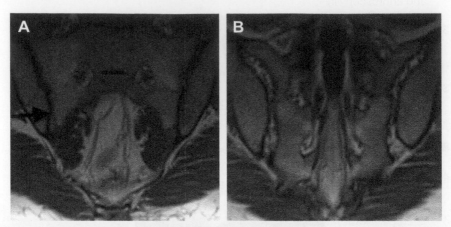

Fig. 2. Normal SIJs. Coronal T1 images through (*A*) the anterior aspect of the joint demonstrating the inferior synovial component (*arrow*) and (*B*) the posterior syndesmotic part.

The standard imaging protocol of the spine and SIJ includes the following:

- Anterior posterior (AP) and lateral views of the cervical, thoracic, and lumbar spines.
- If instability of the cervical spine is suspected, flexion and extension views can be added.
- The SIJs are imaged in true AP (with 30–35° cranial angulation of the tube).
- Oblique views (25–30° posterior angulation of patient) are not frequently requested because it was concluded that AP views alone are satisfactory in more than 85% of the cases as compared with AP pelvis and oblique views combined.[7]

MRI

MRI has become a valuable tool in evaluating inflammatory changes within the axial skeleton. The multiplanar imaging, excellent anatomic detail and tissue contrast, and the ability to modify the imaging sequences have made it preferable to other imaging modalities. The sensitivity and specificity of MRI in detecting early inflammatory changes are far superior to other imaging modalities with a specificity of about 97%.[8]

The routinely used sequences are sagittal T1 and short tau inversion recovery or T2-fat-saturated (T2FS) sequences of the spine (**Fig. 3**) and axial and coronal oblique T1 and T2FS of the sacroiliac joints.

The use of contrast (gadolinium-DTPA) was shown to be superior to T2FS in the detection of active sacroiliitis,[9,10] although T2FS or short tau inversion recovery is usually sufficient in most instances and gadolinium may be used in rare, equivocal cases.[11,12]

Other Imaging Modalities

Computed tomography (CT) demonstrates superior evaluation of sacroiliitis when compared with plain radiography (**Fig. 4**).[13] However, since the advent of MRI with its higher sensitivity and specificity (100% and 94.3%, respectively) and lack of radiation, CT has been of limited value in SpA imaging.[14]

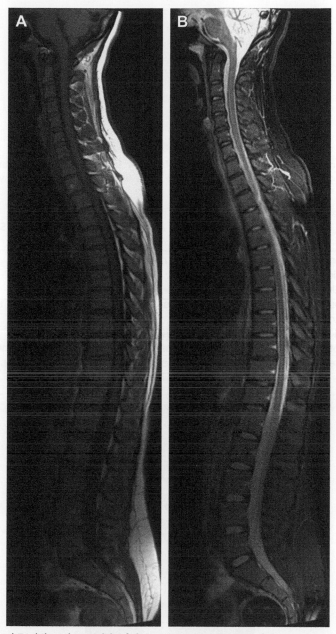

Fig. 3. Sagittal T1 (*A*) and T2FS (*B*) of the entire spine as part of the routine inflammatory protocol demonstrate normal morphology and signal intensity of the vertebrae, discs, and ligamentous structures.

Scintigraphy has a very limited role in the evaluation of inflammatory SpAs,[15,16] while ultrasound has been used to evaluate structural and inflammatory changes at enthyseal insertions, but mainly within the peripheral joints and can differentiate findings related to RA from other SpAs.[17]

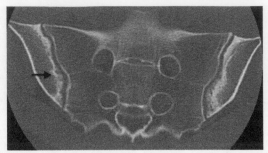

Fig. 4. Coronal reconstructed CT image of bilateral sacroiliitis clearly demarcating the erosive changes along the iliac margins of the joints (*arrow*) with reactive bony sclerosis.

APPROACH TO EVALUATION OF THE SPINE AND SIJS IN INFLAMMATORY SPAS
Spine

1. Bone density: relatively preserved in all disease, except RA (**Fig. 5**)
2. Distribution:
   a. RA: almost exclusively affects the cervical spine
   b. AS, psoriasis, and reactive SpA: initial involvement is at the lumbar spine/thoracolumbar junction
3. Size and shape of vertebral body: squaring in AS
4. Phytes of the spine: these areas of ossification seen at or close to the vertebral body are observed in many diseases that may affect the spine, including

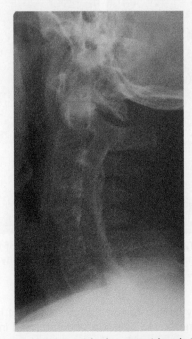

Fig. 5. Severe osteopenia in a patient with rheumatoid arthritis. Note the diffuse facet ankylosis.

degenerative joint disease. There are 4 types of phytes described in the literature. Detecting the type of phyte is important in diagnosing the type of arthropathy:

a. Syndesmophytes: ossification of Sharpey fibers and the deep fibers of the ALL (**Fig. 6**A), which appear as a smooth vertical ossification that connects 2 vertebral bodies across the disc space. AS is the prototype of such phytes, which may also be seen in reactive, psoriatic, or enteropathic arthropathies.

b. Marginal osteophytes: horizontal projections at the level of the vertebral endplate, with its cortex and medulla continuous with those of the parent bone (see **Fig. 6**B). If large, they may become vertical and join another marginal phyte at an adjacent level and are usually seen in degenerative joint disease (DJD) or posttraumatic conditions.

c. Nonmarginal osteophytes (tractional osteophytes): about 2 to 3 mm away from the endplate, are also continuous with the cortex and medulla, and start horizontally but may become vertical as in the marginal ones (see **Fig. 6**C). Smaller phytes are seen in DJD or spondylosis deformans; however, larger ones (also called nonmarginal syndesmophytes) are seen in psoriatic and reactive arthritis.

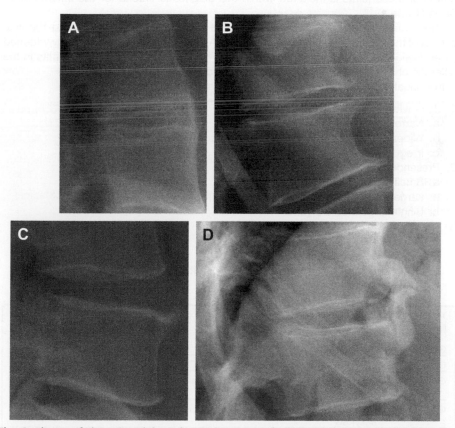

Fig. 6. Phytes of the spine: (*A*) syndesmophytes—ossification of the annulus fibrosus, (*B*) marginal osteophytes, arising from the endplate, (*C*) nonmarginal osteophytes, arising 2 to 3 mm away from the endplate, (*D*) paraspinal phytes, arising outside the discovertebral complex, usually ALL ossification.

    d. Paraspinal phytes: Ossification of structures outside the vertebral body or disc, usually the ALL (see **Fig. 6**D). The ossification is separated from the vertebral body by a thin, lucent cleft. This pattern is normally associated with diffuse idiopathic skeletal hyperostosis.

5. Distribution of phytes:
    a. AS: symmetric and confluent and usually starts from lumbar spine
    b. Psoriatic/reactive: asymmetric and demonstrates a skip distribution[18]

6. The intervertebral disc:
    a. Calcification: classically seen in calcium pyrophosphate deposition disease (CPPD), but may be seen in later stages of AS

Pearl: Commonest Cause of Discal Calcification Is Osteoarthritis

7. Height:
    a. Maintained in AS and psoriatic/reactive arthritis
    b. Narrowed in DJD, CPPD, and ochronosis (alkaptonurea)

Sacroiliac Joints

The SIJs are commonly affected by inflammatory arthropathies, and the imaging evaluation of these joints is included within the diagnostic criteria for the inflammatory SpAs (**Table 1**).[19]

    The earliest observed changes are loss of the cortical white line along the iliac aspect of the joint followed by erosions (**Fig. 7**A). The joint may appear initially widened (pseudowidening). In an attempt to heal, new bone is deposited, which results in the sclerotic changes, eventually leading to ankylosis (see **Fig. 7**B).

    In evaluating the SIJs, the following points are considered:

1. Joint width:
    a. Narrow: RA
    b. Wide: infection and seropositive SpAs
    c. Irregular: DJD, CPPD

2. Presence and type of erosions:
    a. Small and succinct: AS and RA
    b. Large and extensive: psoriatic, reactive, septic arthritis
    c. Single large erosion: gout

3. Presence and type of sclerotic changes:
    a. Minimal: AS
    b. Extensive: psoriatic, reactive, septic
    c. Triangular and only on the iliac sides: osteitis condensans Ilii.

Table 1	
New York criteria for inflammatory sacroiliitis	
Grade 0	Normal
Grade 1	Suspicious changes
Grade 2	Minimal definite changes: circumscribed areas with erosions or sclerosis with no changes of the sacroiliac joint space
Grade 3	Distinctive changes, sclerosis, change of joint space (decrease or widened), partial ankylosis
Grade 4	Ankylosis

From Moll JM, Wright V. New York clinical criteria for ankylosing spondylitis. A statistical evaluation. Ann Rheum Dis 1973;32(4):354–63; with permission.

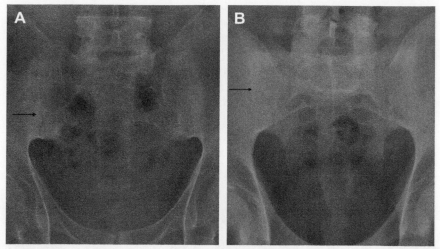

Fig. 7. Inflammatory sacroiliitis. (*A*) Bilateral grade (3): erosions, sclerosis, and narrowing (*arrow*). (*B*) Bilateral grade (4): completely ankylosed SIJs in a patient with AS (*arrow*).

4. Presence and type of bony bridging:
   a. Only the synovial portion: RA
   b. The entire SIJ: all the other inflammatory arthropathies and infection
5. Distribution of changes:
   a. Unilateral: infection
   b. Bilateral symmetric: AS, enteropathic arthritis, CPPD
   c. Bilateral asymmetric: psoriatic and reactive arthritis and gout[18,20]

IMAGING FINDINGS IN SPECIFIC DISEASE ENTITIES
Axial Spondyloarthritis

Ankylosing spondylitis
AS is an inflammatory disease of unknown cause that is linked to HLA-B27. It affects about 0.1% of the population and men are affected more than women. Disease onset is during the second to fourth decades of life. It initially affects the thoracolumbar/lumbosacral junctions, but eventually involves the entire spine.[21]

Spinal involvement
- Discovertebral unit:
  o Erosive changes along the superior and inferior corners of the vertebral bodies: osteitis—also named Romano lesions
  o Bone laying in an attempt to repair will lead to vertebral body squaring (loss of the anterior concavity) and shiny corners (**Fig. 8**)
  o Syndesmophytes: smooth and bilateral will predominate along the anterior and lateral aspects of the vertebral bodies, and when extensive, will produce the characteristic "Bamboo spine" (**Fig. 9**).
  o Erosions and destruction: although not a prominent part of AS, erosions may occur along the central or peripheral aspects of the endplate. Destruction of the discovertebral junction of 2 adjacent vertebrae is characteristic of AS.
  o Discal calcification

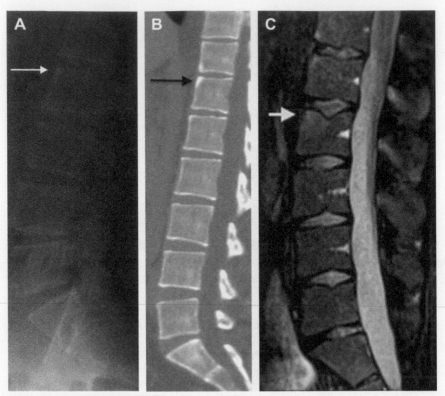

Fig. 8. The appearance of shiny corners on a lateral lumbar spine radiograph (*A*) and a sagittal reconstruction of a lumbar spine CT (*B*) demonstrate sclerotic changes along the corners of the vertebral bodies (*arrow*). (*C*) Sagittal T2FS MRI of the lumbar spine reveals high signal in keeping with marrow edema (*arrow*).

- ○ Disc ballooning: biconcave appearance of vertebral body, especially with osteoporosis, will lead to discal ballooning (**Fig. 10**)
- Apophyseal joints: erosions and sclerosis
  - ○ Bony ankylosis: occurs following ankylosis of the apophyseal joints and capsular ossification across the discs[22]
  - ○ Ligamentous attachments: may develop calcification, ossification, and subligamentous erosions. Ossification of the posterior interspinous ligament results in the "dagger sign" and the fused facets along with the ligamentous ossification account for the "trolley track sign."[23]
  - ○ The early inflammatory changes within the ligaments may present as edema characterized by increased T2 signal on MRI (**Fig. 11**).

Sacroiliac joints

- Bilateral and symmetric with small erosions
- Not significant sclerosis
- Ankylosis early in disease and affects synovial and fibrocartilagenous parts of the joint as well as the surrounding ligaments (**Fig. 12**)

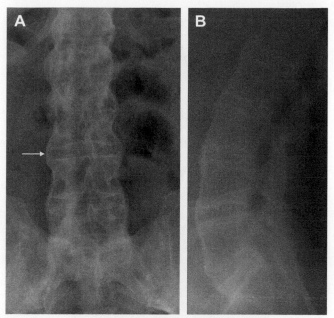

Fig. 9. AP (*A*) and lateral (*B*) views of the lumbar spine in an AS patient. Complete ossification of the annulus fibrosus (*arrow* in *A*) resulting in a bamboo spine. Note the SIJ ankylosis on the AP and the vertebral body squaring on the lateral views.

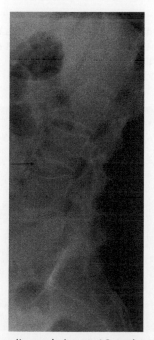

Fig. 10. Lateral lumbar spine radiograph in an AS patient with disc ballooning (*arrow*) secondary to biconcave appearance of the vertebral bodies.

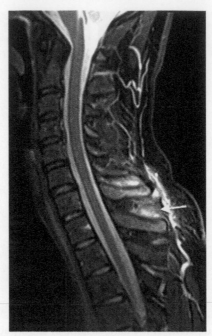

Fig. 11. Sagittal T2FS MRI of the cervical spine in a patient with AS with striking edema within the interspinous ligaments (*arrow*) in keeping with inflammatory changes. Again, squaring of the cervical vertebrae is evident.

Complications

- Atlantoaxial instability with neurologic symptoms is unusual
- Cord compression, in the lumbar region as a result of spondylodiscitis
- Fractures and pseudoarthrosis
- Spinal canal stenosis and cauda equina syndrome

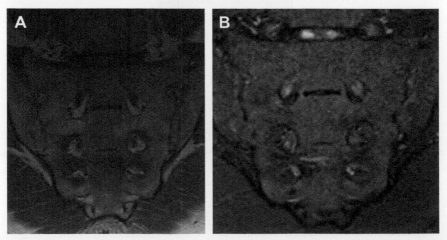

Fig. 12. Coronal T1 (*A*) and T2FS (*B*) of the SIJs demonstrate complete ankylosis in a patient with AS.

Pitfalls

- Ochronosis, a rare autosomal-recessive disorder, demonstrates discal calcification along the annulus fibrosis that may resemble the bamboo spine of AS; however, the diffuse disc height reduction, vaccum phenomena, and gross degenerative changes are against AS. Also the SIJ may demonstrate degenerative changes but will not fuse.[24]
- Scheuermann disease: an osteochondrosis involving the thoracic and thoracolumbar endplates may be clinically confused for AS. The endplate irregularity, the anterior wedging of the adjacent vertebral bodies with a subsequent kyphotic deformity, isdiagnostic (**Fig. 13**).[25]

Psoriatic and reactive arthritis

Psoriatic arthritis (PsA) is an immune-mediated disorder that affects multiple organs and may affect the skeleton in 10% to 15% of patients with skin manifestations.[23] Its age of onset is less than 40 years.

Reactive arthritis is a sterile arthritis that occurs as a response to infection elsewhere in the body, with the classical triad of arthritis, conjunctivitis, and urethritis (or cervicitis). The spinal involvement of both diseases is very similar and is described simultaneously.

Spinal involvement

- Discovertebral unit
  - Erosive changes may occur along the endplates and may be associated with spondylodiscitis

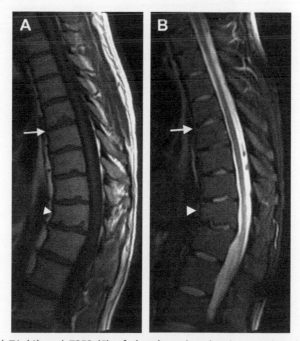

Fig. 13. Sagittal T1 (*A*) and T2FS (*B*) of the thoracic spine in a patient initially thought to have AS. MRI revealed endplate irregularity (*white arrows*) and kyphotic deformity (*arrowheads*) within the lower thoracic spine in keeping with Scheuermann disease.

- ○ The osteophytes are usually bulky and nonmarginal. They are usually asymmetric with skip areas (**Fig. 14**).[26]
- ○ Reparative bony changes are excuberant (**Fig. 15**).
- Apophyseal joints: involved in the cervical spine, with erosive changes, sclerosis, and ankylosis. Cervical spine changes are usually the most severe.[27]

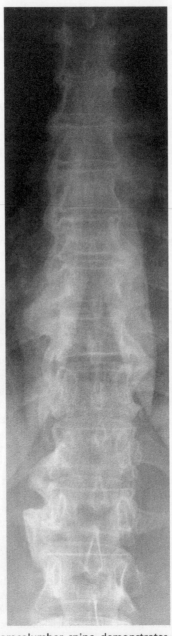

Fig. 14. AP view of the thoracolumbar spine demonstrates bulky, asymmetric phytes in a patient with PsA.

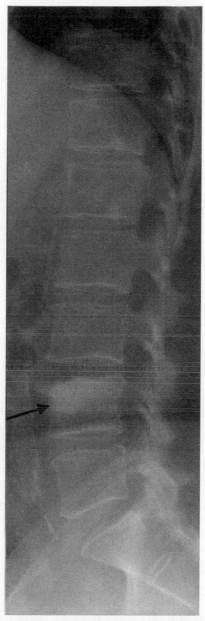

Fig. 15. Endplate sclerosis in another patient with PsA demonstrating the excuberant bone repair (*arrow*).

- Bony ankylosis: occasionally occurs across the apophyseal joints of the cervical spine. Disc height is usually maintained
- Enthesitis around the axial and appendicular skeleton is a common finding (**Fig. 16**)[28]
- Spinal changes are commoner in PsA than in reactive arthritis

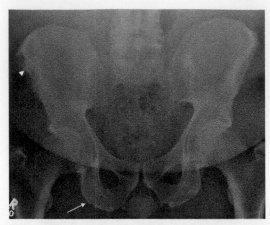

Fig. 16. AP view of the pelvis in a psoriatic patient with enthesopathic changes within the anterior superior iliac spine (*arrowhead*) and ischial tuberosities (*white arrow*).

Sacroiliac joints

- Initially unilateral and may mimic infection
- Becomes bilateral and asymmetrical
- Erosions are larger than the ones seen in AS and RA
- Profound sclerosis
- Ankylosis uncommon
- SIJ ligaments can ossify before ankylosis occurs

Complications

- Atlantoaxial instability as a result of the cervical spine facet joint erosions

Pitfall: the bulky paraspinal phytes of diffuse idiopathic skeletal hyperostosis may be confused for PsA; however, the preserved disc spaces, and lack of apophyseal or SIJ abnormalities exclude an underlying inflammatory cause.

Enteropathic arthritis

Enteropathic arthritis is another SpA with HLA-B27 association. It occurs in patients with inflammatory bowel disease, and Whipple disease, with spondylitis and sacroiliitis similar to AS. It should be suspected in young patients with bilateral symmetric sacroiliitis and symptoms and signs of bowel disease or bowel surgery (**Fig. 17**).[29]

Seropositive Arthritis

Rheumatoid arthritis

RA is a chronic condition affecting about 0.5% to 1% of the population. It affects women 2 to 3 times more than men and predominates between 25 and 55 years of age. Several genetic as well as environmental causes are suggested as causative factors.[30] The rheumatoid factor is positive in about 75% of the patients.[31]

The disease is a symmetric inflammatory arthropathy that primarily involves the synovial joints of the peripheral skeleton, but can also involve the spine, in particular, the cervical vertebra, and can result in potentially life-threatening complications.

Spinal involvement

Involvement of the cervical spine is as high as 85%.

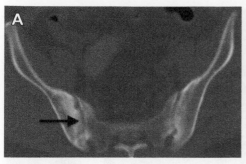 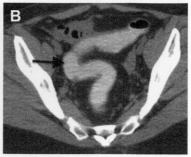

Fig. 17. Bone window of a CT scan through the sacroiliac joints (*A*) demonstrates bilateral grade 3 sacroiliitis (*arrow*). (*B*) Soft tissue window through the pelvis demonstrates an ahaustral colon (*arrow*). Findings in keeping with enteropathic arthritis.

- Occipitoatlantoaxial articulations
  - ○ Atlantoaxial (AA) subluxation
    - ▪ Anteroposterior AA subluxation: one of the earliest abnormalities, which occurs in 20% to 25% of the patients and is defined as a distance of more than 2.5 mm between the posterior aspect of the atlas and the anterior aspect of the axis (usually measured along the inferior aspect of the articulation) (**Fig. 18**). It is thought to be related to transverse ligament laxity.
    - ▪ Vertical AA subluxation: also called cranial settling and atlantoaxial impaction, occurs when the osseous, cartilaginous, or ligamentous structures between the occiput, atlas, and axis become disrupted, resulting in superior migration of the dens or inferior migration of the cranium.[32,33] Several lines have been used to measure the distances between C1, C2, and the occiput, but, in general, crowding of the structures in this area and also displacement of the dens beyond foramen magnum are features to look for on a lateral radiograph (**Fig. 19**).

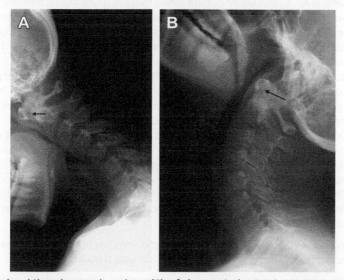

Fig. 18. Flexion (*A*) and extension views (*B*) of the cervical spine in an RA patient demonstrate an increased atlantoaxial interval on flexion that is reduced on extension (*arrows*), in keeping with AP atlantoaxial instability.

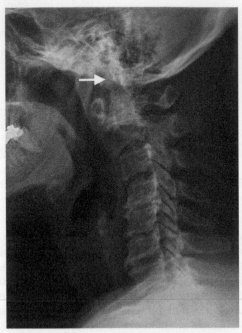

Fig. 19. Lateral radiograph of the cervical spine in another RA patient. There is widening of the atlantodens interval in keeping with anterior AA subluxation. There is also superior migration of the dens, with its tip a few millimeters above the foramen magnum (*arrow*), in keeping with cranial settling.

- Lateral AA subluxation: occurs when there is more than 2 mm displacement between the lateral masses of the atlas and the axis on an AP plain film. It usually occurs because of articular space narrowing, bone erosion, and disruption of the articular capsules followed by collapse of the lateral masses in severe cases.
- Subaxial subluxations: occurs in 9% of patients with chronic disease and commonly affects multiple levels, producing a "stepladder" or "doorstep" appearance, with anterior subluxation more common than posterior. If localized, it is more common at C3-4 and C4-5.
- Odontoid erosions: occur in 14% to 35% of patients as a result of chronic synovial inflammation. Pathologic fractures may occur. The odontoid process may be significantly reduced in size (**Fig. 20**).
- Apophyseal joints: osteopenia, narrowing, and superficial erosions.
- Discovertebral joints and joints of Luschka: disc space narrowing, osseous irregularity, eburnation, and superficial erosions in the absence of osteophytes. Multiple levels are affected.

The findings in relation to the apophyseal and discovertebral joints may be observed in the thoracic and lumbar spine, although much less frequent.

- Spinous process erosions and destruction in the lower cervical/upper thoracic spine lead to sharp spinous processes that may lead to inflammatory changes within the supraspinatous ligaments.

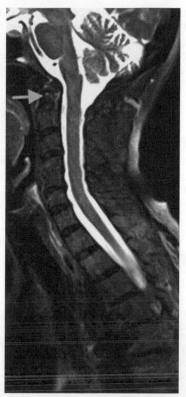

Fig. 20. Sagittal T2FS MRI image of the cervical spine in an RA patient. The odontoid process is severely reduced in size (*arrow*) in keeping with erosions. It is also superiorly migrated and is at the level of the clivus.

Sacroiliac joints

- Infrequent and mild, affecting 25% to 35% of patients with severe longstanding disease
- Bilateral but not necessarily symmetric
- Erosions superficial and well-marginated
- Ankylosis occurs later in the disease and only affects synovial portion

Complications

- Compression of bulbomedullary and cranial nerves, spinal and vertebral arteries, and hydrocephalus as a result of vertical subluxation
- Myelopathy related to subaxial subluxation (although rare)
- Avascular necrosis and insufficiency fractures related to treatment[22]

Pearls and pitfalls of RA

- Careful observation of the upper cervical spine to detect early instability. If subluxation was not visualized on the routine lateral C-spine view, flexion views can detect instability at the atlantoaxial and subaxial levels.

- The presence of odontoid tip erosions may prevent the diagnosis of vertical subluxation. Always look for the relationship between the occiput, C1, and C2. Is there any crowding of the structures?
- Multilevel discovertebral endplate changes with sclerosis in the absence of osteophytes raises the possibility of RA rather than degenerative disc disease.

DIFFERENTIAL DIAGNOSIS AND POTENTIAL PITFALLS INVOLVING THE SPINE AND SACROILIAC JOINTS
CPPD Crystal Deposition Disease

Chondrocalcinosis of the annulus fibrosus and the SIJs, ossification of the ALL, severe degenerative disc and endplate changes, and tumorlike masses at the atlantoaxial level are characteristics of CPPD (**Fig. 21**).

Infective Spondylodiscitis

Infection may be difficult to differentiate from inflammatory changes, in particular, early in the disease. Certain findings support infection (**Fig. 22**, **Table 2**).[34,35]

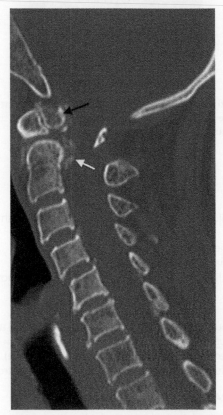

Fig. 21. Sagittal reconstructed image of a cervical spine CT in a patient with CPPD. Calcified mass is noted surrounding the atlantoaxial joint (*white arrow*) with subluxation of an os-odontium (*black arrow*).

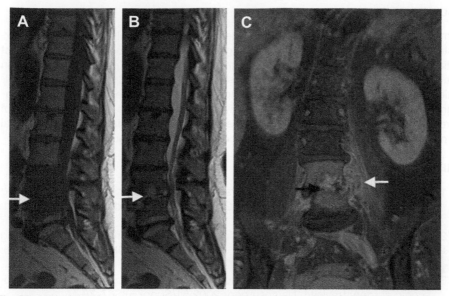

Fig. 22. MRI of the lumbar spine. (*A*) Sagittal T1 demonstrates diffuse signal abnormality of L4 and L5 vertebrae and the intervening disc (*arrow*). (*B*) Sagittal T2 shows an increased signal within the disc and the endplates (*arrow*). (*C*) Postcontrast coronal T1FS demonstrates diffuse enhancement of the L4–5 disc and the adjacent vertebrae with enhancement of the paravertebral soft tissues (*arrows*) in keeping with infective spondylodiscitis.

Axial Neuropathic Arthropathy

Axial neuropathic arthropathy may occur in syphilis, diabetes, and syringomyelia. The radiographic findings may resemble osteoarthritis but appear more aggressive.

Initial changes: disc height loss, end-plate sclerosis

- Later: increased sclerosis, subluxations, fragmentation, and bizarre osteophytosis[22]
- On MRI, the changes are characteristically low on T1 and T2[36]

Table 2
Findings on plain film and MRI suggestive of spinal infection

Modality	Plain Film	MRI
	Osteopenia (TB)	Vertebral edema
	Endplate irregularity followed by height reduction and destruction	Endplate erosion or destruction (T1 or T2)
	Disc space narrowing	Disc height reduction with T2 hyperintensity and postcontrast enhancement
	Paraspinal soft tissue mass	Paraspinal ± epidural mass
	Reactive sclerosis (late)	
	SIJ: ill-defined, blurry margins	SIJ: edema, irregularity, joint effusion, or fluid collection

SUMMARY

Imaging of the spine is an everyday challenge to the radiologist. A thorough understanding of the natural history and the imaging findings is indispensable to the correct diagnosis. Developing an approach to image evaluation, in particular of the plain radiograph, will lead to the correct diagnosis in most instances. Other imaging modalities, especially MRI, have been increasingly used in the earlier phases when radiographs are negative, and therefore, play an important role in early initiation of treatment. It also plays an important role when the clinical findings are equivocal and other disease entities affecting the spine are to be ruled out.

REFERENCES

1. Linden SV, Valkenburg HA, Cats A. Evaluation of diagnostic criteria for ankylosing spondylitis. Arthritis Rheum 1984;27(4):361–8. http://dx.doi.org/10.1002/art.1780270401.
2. Beckingsale AB, Davies J, Gibson JM, et al. Acute anterior uveitis, ankylosing spondylitis, back pain, and HLA-B27. Br J Ophthalmol 1984;68(10):741–5. http://dx.doi.org/10.1136/bjo.68.10.741.
3. Pait TG, Elias AJ, Tribell R. Thoracic, lumbar, and sacral spine anatomy for endoscopic surgery [review]. Neurosurgery 2002;51(Suppl 5):S67–78.
4. Modic MT, Masaryk TJ, Ross JS, et al. Imaging of degenerative disk disease. Radiology 1988;168:177–86.
5. Mester AR, Makó EK, Karlinger K, et al. Enteropathic arthritis in the sacroiliac joint. Imaging and differential diagnosis. Eur J Radiol 2000;35(3):199–208. http://dx.doi.org/10.1016/S0720-048X(00)00243-6A.
6. Sieper J. Developments in therapies for spondyloarthritis. Nat Rev Rheumatol 2012;8(5):280–7. http://dx.doi.org/10.1038/nrrheum.2012.40.
7. Battistone MJ, Manaster BJ, Reda DJ, et al. Radiographic diagnosis of sacroiliitis–are sacroiliac views really better? J Rheumatol 1998;25(12):2395–401.
8. Weber U, Maksymowych WP. Sensitivity and specificity of magnetic resonance imaging for axial spondyloarthritis. Am J Med Sci 2011;341(4):272–7. http://dx.doi.org/10.1097/MAJ.0b013e31820f8c59.
9. Althoff CE, Feist E, Burova E, et al. Magnetic resonance imaging of active sacroiliitis: do we really need gadolinium? Eur J Radiol 2009;71(2):232–6. http://dx.doi.org/10.1016/j.ejrad.2009.04.034.
10. Bollow M, Braun J, Hamm B, et al. Early sacroiliitis in patients with spondyloarthropathy: evaluation with dynamic gadolinium-enhanced MR imaging. Radiology 1995;194(2):529–36.
11. Rostom S, Dougados M, Gossec L. New tools for diagnosing spondyloarthropathy. Joint Bone Spine 2010;77(2):108–14. http://dx.doi.org/10.1016/j.jbspin.2009.12.005.
12. Canella C, Schau B, Ribeiro E, et al. MRI in seronegative spondyloarthritis: imaging features and differential diagnosis in the spine and sacroiliac joints [review]. AJR Am J Roentgenol 2013;200:149–57. http://dx.doi.org/10.2214/AJR.12.8858.
13. Fam AG, Rubenstein JD, Chin-Sang H, et al. Computed tomography in the diagnosis of early ankylosing spondylitis. Arthritis Rheum 1985;28(8):930–7. http://dx.doi.org/10.1002/art.1780280813.
14. Wittram C, Whitehouse GH, Williams JW, et al. Comparison of MR and CT in suspected sacroiliitis. J Comput Assist Tomogr 1996;20(1):68.
15. Song IH, Carrasco-Fernández J, Rudwaleit M. The diagnostic value of scintigraphy in assessing sacroiliitis in ankylosing spondylitis: a systematic literature research. Ann Rheum Dis 2008;67(11):1535–40.

16. Rau R, Wasserberg S, Backhaus M. Imaging methods in rheumatology: imaging in psoriasis arthritis (PsA). Z Rheumatol 2006;65(2):159–67.

17. D'Agostino MA. Ultrasound imaging in spondyloarthropathies. Best Pract Res Clin Rheumatol 2010;24(5):693–700. http://dx.doi.org/10.1016/j.berh.2010.05.003.

18. Brower AC, Flemming DJ. Arthritis in black and white. 3rd edition. Philadelphia: Elsevier/Saunders; 2012. ISBN-13: 978-1-4160-5595-2.

19. Moll JM, Wright V. New York clinical criteria for ankylosing spondylitis. A statistical evaluation. Ann Rheum Dis 1973;32(4):354–63.

20. Grigoryan M, Roemer FW, Mohr A, et al. Imaging in spondyloarthropathies. Curr Rheumatol Rep 2004;6(2):102–9. http://dx.doi.org/10.1007/s11926-004-0054-8.

21. Jang JH, Ward MM, Rucker AN, et al. Ankylosing spondylitis: patterns of radiographic involvement–a re-examination of accepted principles in a cohort of 769 patients. Radiology 2010;258(1):192–8. http://dx.doi.org/10.1148/radiol.10100426.

22. Resnick D, Kransdorf MJ. Bone and joint imaging. 3rd edition. Elsevier; 2005. ISBN-10: 072160270.

23. Jacobson JA, Girish G, Jiang Y, et al. Radiographic evaluation of arthritis: inflammatory conditions. Radiology 2008;248(2):378–89. http://dx.doi.org/10.1148/radiol.

24. Balaban B, Taskaynatan M, Yasar E, et al. Ochronotic spondyloarthropathy: spinal involvement resembling ankylosing spondylitis. Clin Rheumatol 2005; 25(4):598–601. http://dx.doi.org/10.1007/s10067-005-0038-8.

25. Paajanen H, Alanen A, Erkintalo M, et al. Disc degeneration in Scheuermann disease. Skeletal Radiol 1989;18(7):523–6.

26. McQueen F, Lassere M. Magnetic resonance imaging in psoriatic arthritis: a review of the literature. Arthritis Res Ther 2006;8(2):207.

27. Helliwell PS, Hickling P, Wright V. Do the radiological changes of classic ankylosing spondylitis differ from the changes found in the spondylitis associated with inflammatory bowel disease, psoriasis, and reactive arthritis? Ann Rheum Dis 1998;57(3):135–40. http://dx.doi.org/10.1136/ard.57.3.135.

28. McGonagle D, Gibbon W, Emery P. Classification of inflammatory arthritis by enthesitis. Lancet 1998;352(9134):1137–40. http://dx.doi.org/10.1016/S0140-6736(97) 12004-9.

29. Björkengren AG, Resnick D, Sartoris DJ. Enteropathic arthropathies. Radiol Clin North Am 1987;25(1):189–98.

30. Doran MF, Pond GR, Crowson CS, et al. Trends in incidence and mortality in rheumatoid arthritis in Rochester, Minnesota, over a forty-year period. Arthritis Rheum 2002;46(3):625–31. http://dx.doi.org/10.1002/art.509.

31. Withrington RH, Teitsson I, Valdimarsson H, et al. Prospective study of early rheumatoid arthritis. II. Association of rheumatoid factor isotypes with fluctuations in disease activity. Ann Rheum Dis 1984;43(5):679–85. http://dx.doi.org/10.1136/ard.43.5.679.

32. Halla JT, Hardin JG, Vitek J, et al. Involvement of the cervical spine in rheumatoid arthritis. Arthritis Rheum 1989;32(5):652–9. http://dx.doi.org/10.1002/anr.17803 20522.

33. El-Khoury GY, Wener MH, Menezes AH, et al. Cranialsettling in rheumatoid arthritis. Radiology 1980;137(3):637–42.

34. Tyrrell PN, Cassar-Pullicino VN, McCall IW. Spinal infection. Eur Radiol 1999;9(6): 1066–77. http://dx.doi.org/10.1007/s003300050793.

35. Ledermann HP, Schweitzer ME, Morrison WB, et al. MR imaging findings in spinal infections: rules or myths? Radiology 2003;228(2):506–14. http://dx.doi.org/ 10.1148/radiol.2282020752.

36. Park YH, Taylor JA, Szollar SM, et al. Imaging findings in spinal neuroarthropathy. Spine 1994;19(13):1499–504.

Ultrasound and Treatment Algorithms of RA and JIA

Sam R. Dalvi, MD[a], David W. Moser, DO[b],
Jonathan Samuels, MD[a],*

KEYWORDS

- Rheumatoid arthritis • Juvenile idiopathic arthritis • Musculoskeletal ultrasound

KEY POINTS

- Musculoskeletal ultrasound has emerged as a key tool for the diagnosis, prognosis, and management of patients with RA (rheumatoid arthritis) and other rheumatic diseases.
- The most important sonographic findings in RA include erosions, effusions, synovitis, and tenosynovitis.
- Investigators have suggested various "optimal" numbers of joints to scan in RA to assess disease activity, gauge treatment response, provide prognostic information, and guide management decisions.
- The complexity of pediatric sonoanatomy has delayed its validation in juvenile idiopathic arthritis, yet ultrasound reliably measures the extent of synovitis/tenosynovitis and guides precise injections.

INTRODUCTION

The field of rheumatology has made great strides over the past 2 decades in understanding the pathogenesis of rheumatoid arthritis (RA), as well as developing biologic treatments that have fundamentally altered the natural history of the disease. These emerging therapeutic options in part spurred the 2010 update of the RA classification (and diagnostic) criteria,[1] which stresses the importance of early identification and aggressive treatment of RA, not only for alleviating symptoms but also for altering the disease process and preventing damage. Yet these criteria, as well as measures of disease activity (HAQ-DI, DAS-28) and serum markers of inflammation (erythrocyte sedimentation rate [ESR] and C-reactive protein [CRP]), often are not sufficiently reliable in identifying patients with RA or assessing their disease activity.[2–5] Moreover, these tests are oftentimes difficult for patients to understand in meaningful ways.

Perhaps addressing these shortcomings, rheumatologists overseas (and more recently in the United States) have increasingly looked to musculoskeletal ultrasound

---

[a] Division of Rheumatology, Center for Musculoskeletal Care, NYU Langone Medical Center, 333 East 38th Street, 4th Floor. New York, NY 10016, USA; [b] Dell Children's Hospital Medical Center, 4900 Mueller Boulevard, Austin, TX 78723, USA
* Corresponding author.
E-mail address: Jonathan.samuels@nyumc.org

Rheum Dis Clin N Am 39 (2013) 669–688
http://dx.doi.org/10.1016/j.rdc.2013.02.015
0889-857X/13/$ – see front matter © 2013 Elsevier Inc. All rights reserved.

(MSUS) to aid in the diagnosis and management of RA and other types of arthritis. Although other imaging modalities provide helpful information about RA, MSUS holds many advantages over plain radiography and magnetic resonance imaging (MRI), and can be performed during the clinical visit by ultrasound-trained rheumatologists (**Box 1**).[6] Not only can MSUS aid in the diagnosis of RA in difficult cases, but many studies have demonstrated that it can provide prognostic insight and have implications for treatment decisions. For instance, a 2008 study by Brown and colleagues[7] (presented later in more detail) identified patients in clinical "remission" with subclinical inflammation by MSUS that predicted ongoing structural damage. In their study, the conventional measures of disease activity often lacked sensitivity to identify the need for more aggressive treatment, whereas the presence of synovitis, as defined by MSUS, was highly associated with progressive radiographic changes.

As the excitement about MSUS has spread to other disorders within rheumatology, assisting in the diagnosis and treatment of crystal disease, spondyloarthropathies, osteoarthritis, and others, the most robust and organized investigations appear in the RA and juvenile idiopathic arthritis (JIA) literature. The results of these studies have, in many ways, ushered in a Renaissance in rheumatology, questioning previously "accepted" methods of examination and changing the way rheumatologists think about arthritic disease. We will show that in the past 5 years, sonographers have proposed various MSUS scoring systems for use in RA research studies and in clinical practice, yet a gold standard consensus for using this imaging modality in RA treatment algorithms remains elusive.

HISTORICAL PERSPECTIVE OF MSUS IN RHEUMATOID ARTHRITIS

One of the earliest reported cases of a patient with RA evaluated by using MSUS was a 1972 report of a patient with a large Baker's cyst, which was clinically diagnosed as thrombophlebitis.[8] In 1978, Cooperberg and colleagues[9] speculated on the usefulness of MSUS in RA by its ability to better characterize suprapatellar effusion sizes, popliteal cysts, and synovial thickening. It was not until the 1990s that the body of literature evaluating RA with MSUS began to expand. A 1993 study by Grassi and colleagues[10] identified significant sonographic findings in RA (described later in more detail), including erosions, synovitis, and joint effusions. In 1995, Lund and colleagues[11] also described the articular abnormalities of the metacarpophalangeal (MCP) as well as carpal joints in 29 patients with RA and were able to correlate these findings with disease severity based on clinical assessment.

Although studies demonstrated the ability of MSUS to identify both articular and periarticular disease in RA, subsequent efforts were aimed at comparing MSUS with

---

Box 1
Advantages of musculoskeletal ultrasound

No complications

No ionizing radiation

No claustrophobia, anxiety, or need for sedation or anesthesia

No contraindications (metal implants or pacemakers)

Ability to generate dynamic images

Ability to assess multiple joints in one session

Relatively low cost

Table 1
Features of RA based on imaging modality

	Erosions	Synovitis	Tenosynovitis	Peri-Articular Osteopenia
Radiograph	Yes	No	No	Yes
Magnetic resonance imaging	Yes	Yes	Yes	Yes
Ultrasound	Yes	Yes	Yes	No

clinical examination, conventional radiography, and MRI (**Table 1**). A 1999 prospective study of 60 patients with inflammatory arthritis (36 with RA) looked at MSUS versus plain radiography, bone scintigraphy, and MRI, concluding that both MSUS and MRI were better able to identify both tenosynovitis and erosive changes in patients without apparent radiographic abnormalities.[12] In 2005, Naredo and colleagues[13] studied 94 patients with RA to demonstrate that MSUS was superior to clinical examination in evaluating disease activity in terms of effusions and synovitis, and that the intraobserver/interobserver reliability was similarly more robust with MSUS than with clinical examination. Since then, several other studies have shown similar findings comparing MSUS to clinical examination, and have also shown MSUS to reveal erosions earlier in the disease process than does plain radiography.[14–16] Numerous studies have also found that MSUS can usually detect erosions and synovitis, as well as (and sometimes better than) the more expensive and less accessible MRI tests (**Table 2**).[17,18] One report by Swen and colleagues[19] evaluating finger tenosynovitis in 21 patients with RA found that the sensitivity and specificity for the determination of partial tendon tears was slightly higher using MSUS compared with MRI. Although the precise role for MSUS in RA management was not yet defined, these earlier studies at least started the discussion in defining its proper place among other useful imaging modalities in RA.

KEY SONOGRAPHICALLY DEFINED PATHOLOGY IN RA

The identification of certain sonographic features of RA has become particularly useful in both clinical practice and research studies. The salient findings include erosions,

Table 2
Sensitivity/specificity of imaging modalities to detect RA synovitis and erosions

		Synovitis			Erosions	
		Sensitivity (%)	Specificity (%)		Sensitivity (%)	Specificity (%)
Szkudlarek	PE	40	85	XR	42	99
et al,[14] 2006	US	70	78	US	59	98
Wakefield	PE	55–83	23–46		N/A	
et al,[15] 2008	US	64–89	60–80			
Rahmani		N/A		XR	13	100
et al,[16] 2010				US	63	98
Alarcon		N/A		MRI	100	65
et al,[113] 2002				US	100	45

MRI served as the gold standard for all of the studies except the article by Alarcon and colleagues, in which x-ray was the standard.

Abbreviations: MRI, magnetic resonance imaging; N/A, not applicable; PE, physical exam; US, ultrasound; XR, x-ray.

effusions, synovitis, and tenosynovitis. Before 2004, there was a scarcity of both reliability and validity data using MSUS, as well as little consensus around definitions of pathologic findings of inflammatory arthritis. In response to this, a group of international sonographers created the OMERACT Ultrasound Task Force to address these deficiencies.[20] Since then, the task force has succeeded in creating standardized definitions for various pathologic findings, as well as improving reliability in the detection of synovitis.[21]

Erosions

Although erosive changes are not a pathognomonic feature of RA, the ability to detect these lesions in the right setting can help to establish a diagnosis, as well as predict more aggressive disease and worse clinical outcomes, justifying more aggressive therapy. Identification of erosions also facilitates enrollment into studies and contributes to outcome measures. Plain radiography at regular intervals was previously used to detect erosions in RA, but this uniplanar technique misses erosive changes early in disease, and damage in patients with superimposed secondary degenerative changes.[22,23] By contrast, MSUS has been shown to detect erosive changes months or years earlier in the disease process and can visualize articular changes in multiple planes of view.

The OMERACT group defines the sonographic bone erosion in RA as "an intra-articular discontinuity of the bone surface that is visible in 2 perpendicular planes."[20] Although erosions can be visualized in many anatomic locations, the most likely areas for detecting hand erosion formation using MSUS include the ulnar styloid process, radial aspect of the second MCP joint, and ulnar aspect of the fifth MCP joint.[24] Because of limitations in probe positioning, MSUS is less useful in evaluation of the carpal bones.

Several studies have shown the superiority of MSUS in the evaluation of erosions compared with conventional radiography.[14,25,26] A 2000 article by Wakefield and colleagues,[25] evaluating the MCP joints of 100 patients with RA, concluded that MSUS was able to detect 127 erosions in 56% of patients, compared with radiographic detection of 32 erosions in only 17% of patients ($P<.0001$). Of note, a subgroup analysis of patients with early RA (disease duration less than 12 months) revealed that 6.5-fold more erosions were seen using MSUS compared with conventional radiography. Another study by Lopez-Ben and colleagues[26] similarly concluded that MSUS surpassed radiography in the ability to detect more erosions in the hands and feet among patients with RA. Although some may defer to MRI for detecting erosions, many studies have shown that MSUS can detect erosions at a similar rate.[27]

Importantly, high interobserver reliability in the detection of bone erosions using MSUS was observed between an experienced radiologist and a rheumatologist.[28] Similar results were obtained more recently following a study in which a rheumatologist without prior experience in sonography underwent an intensive 4-week training course in MSUS and attained high interobserver rates for detecting bone erosions, as compared with a rheumatologist experienced in MSUS.[29]

Effusions

Although pathologic collections of synovial fluid are seen by MSUS in many diseases, including knee osteoarthritis, they are common in almost any active RA joint, from the small hand and foot interphalangeal joints to the medium-sized wrists and larger shoulders and hips (**Fig. 1**). OMERACT defines sonographic effusions as abnormal hypoechoic (gray) or anechoic (black) intra-articular material that is both displaceable

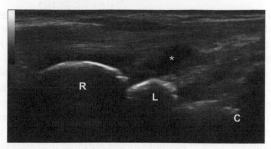

Fig. 1. A 45-year-old woman with longstanding RA currently refusing treatment. Dorsal lon-gitudinal view of the wrist demonstrating an anechoic (*black*) effusion that is compressible on dynamic imaging. The synovial hypertrophy that is also present is not compressible. The bones (*bright white lines*) are labeled: R, radius; L, lunate; C, captitate. The asterisk overlies the effusion.

and compressible, but lacks Doppler signal.[20] MSUS can also quantify the effusion size and assist with both diagnostic and therapeutic arthrocentesis of difficult joints.

Synovitis/Tenosynovitis

OMERACT defines synovial hypertrophy as abnormal hypoechoic intra-articular tissue that is nondisplaceable and poorly compressible, which may exhibit Doppler signal.[30] Proliferative synovitis, also known as pannus, is the hallmark pathologic lesion in RA and represents the primary site of inflammation. Gray-scale images alone for the eval-uation of synovitis (see **Fig. 1**) cannot always discern between acutely and chronically inflamed synovial membranes, as the latter can maintain its thickness over time and make it more difficult to determine therapeutic responses to treatment.[23]

The added information from using power Doppler in addition to the gray-scale imaging information allows the clinician to determine the amount of vascularity within synovial tissue (**Fig. 2**), which can be assessed either semiquantitatively (on a 0–3 scale) or quantitatively (summating pixel numbers in a region of interest).[31] This tech-nique helps assess synovitis in the gamut of joint sizes from the small joints of the digits to the shoulder and hip. In fact, assessment of vascularity using Doppler has been shown to correlate with the histopathologic features of synovitis. A study by Walther and colleagues[32] that evaluated the knee joints of 23 patients with arthritis undergoing arthroplasty showed high correlation (*P*<.01) between Doppler scoring of vascularity performed before surgery and histologic analysis of synovial tissue

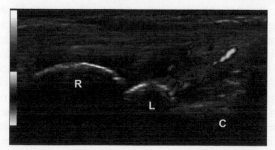

Fig. 2. The same patient with active RA as in **Fig. 1**. Dorsal longitudinal view of the wrist demonstrating synovial hypertrophy and overlying red/yellow power Doppler signal.

(by qualitative and quantitative vessel density in the sample) obtained during the procedure. Another study among patients with severe hip arthritis planning to undergo arthroplasty showed similar results, suggesting that Doppler reliably measures vascularity of synovial tissue.[33]

Ultrasonography is also useful for the detection of tenosynovitis, defined sonographically by OMERACT as either anechoic or hypoechoic tissue with or without fluid in the tendon sheath, seen in 2 perpendicular planes and which may demonstrate Doppler signal.[30] Common locations for tendon involvement in RA are in the hand and wrist, including the flexor digitorum, extensor digitorum (**Fig. 3**), extensor carpi ulnaris, and extensor carpi radialis tendons.[34] Recent studies suggest that evaluation of tenosynovitis using MSUS is reliable, with acceptable intraobserver and interobserver concordance.[35,36]

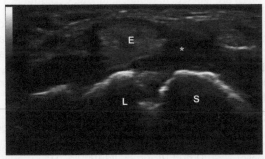

Fig. 3. The same patient with active RA as in **Fig. 1**. Dorsal transverse view of the wrist demonstrating tenosynovitis (*asterisk*) around the extensor tendon (E) superficial to the scaphoid (S) and lunate (L).

KEY PATHOLOGY IN OTHER INFLAMMATORY ARTHRITIDES

Some of the sonographic features seen in RA overlap with those found in other rheumatic diseases, thus it is important to note that they are not pathognomonic for RA. At the same time, some of the other diagnoses have other unique sonographic findings (**Table 3**).

Spondyloarthritides

Although psoriatic arthritis (PsA) and the spondyloarthropathies share some of the RA features detailed previously, both clinically and by ultrasound, evidence of entheseal changes represents one of the major differences, a reflection of its role as an initiating site of injury and subsequent inflammation. Such entheseal inflammation is often subclinical, although estimates of its asymptomatic prevalence in the PsA population vary widely.[37–39] The enthesis represents 1 of the 5 main anatomic structures that can be abnormal sonographically in PsA, with others including the joint, tendon, skin, and nail. One group of investigators who outlined these 5 targets also created a preliminary Doppler score for PsA assessment that involves all 5 of them.[40] Studies have consistently found MSUS to be superior to physical examination and radiograph in the detection of inflammatory changes.[41] The utility of MSUS in management of PsA was demonstrated in a recent retrospective study that suggested that serial Doppler evaluations showed improvements in synovial proliferation and joint effusions (but not bone erosions) during the course of adalimumab therapy.[42] The next step, however, remains the development of an accepted standardized scoring system for PsA assessment.

Table 3
Ultrasound features of various arthritides

Rheumatoid arthritis	Synovitis, effusions, erosions, tenosynovitis
Psoriatic arthritis	Synovitis, effusions, erosions, tenosynovitis, enthesitis[20]
Gout	Synovitis, effusions, erosions, tophi,[48] double contour (uric acid on articular cartilage)[43]
Calcium pyrophosphate disease	Synovitis, effusions, calcium pyrophosphate deposition within articular cartilage, in fibrous cartilage and tendons or as freely mobile nodular deposits in bursae[51]
Osteoarthritis	Synovitis, effusions, osteophytes, articular cartilage thinning[114]

Crystalline Disorders

Although there have been numerous articles outlining the sonographic findings in crystal diseases, they too lack any universal scoring systems. Thiele and Schlesinger[43] identified a "double-contour sign" of urate deposits on the hyaline cartilage in 92% of 23 patients with gout and in none of the control patients diagnosed with other arthritides. Subsequent studies confirmed greater than 98% specificity of the double-contour sign in gout,[44,45] whereas Thiele and Schlesinger[46] later found the double contour to disappear in all 5 patients who achieved a serum urate level less than 6 mg/dL for more than 6 months using urate-lowering drugs. Other investigators have also characterized sonographic findings of tophi and erosions demonstrating better sensitivity versus plain radiography.[47–49] A recent study validated the inter-reader reliability of diagnosing tophi in the first metatarsophalangeal (MTP) joint and a double-contour sign in the femoral articular cartilage in patients with gout and asymptomatic hyperuricemia in a cohort of 75 patients.[50]

MSUS can also detect calcium pyrophosphate disease in a number of different patterns and anatomic locations, including (1) hyperechoic bands within hyaline articular cartilage; (2) punctate hyperechoic spots, more common in fibrous cartilage and tendons; and (3) homogeneous, hyperechoic nodular deposits floating freely within bursae.[51] Although its sensitivity varies widely in the literature, this MSUS finding in chondrocalcinosis appears to be highly specific.[44]

Osteoarthritis

Although osteoarthritis (OA) has long been heralded as a noninflammatory, degenerative disease, MSUS findings are consistent with other clinical and imaging evidence that OA can in fact present with effusions and synovitis (by gray scale and Doppler). Beyond identifying osteophytes and articular cartilage wear, MSUS may serve a prognostic role in these patients. A recent prospective multicenter study of 531 European patients with painful knee OA identified predictive factors for knee replacement, one of which was an MSUS effusion measuring greater than 4 mm (while a clinically apparent effusion was not predictive).[52]

ULTRASOUND SCORING SYSTEMS IN RA

Although MSUS, as shown previously, is able to identify RA disease activity and damage at the "joint" level, many groups have devised methods of scoring at the "patient" level (**Table 4**). Although no single scoring system has demonstrated superiority, the various systems aid in measuring clinical trial outcomes, help the clinician evaluate

Table 4
Comparison of various MSUS joint scoring systems

	No. of Joints	Specific Joints Scanned	What Is Scored[a]	Time Needed
Scirè et al,[56] 2009	44	Bilateral shoulders, elbows, wrists, MCPs, PIPs, sternoclaviculars, acromioclaviculars, knees, ankles, MTPs	Synovitis	About 60 min
Naredo et al,[13] 2005	28	Bilateral MCPs, PIPs, wrists, elbows, shoulders, knees	Effusion, synovitis	Maximum 30 min
Perricone et al,[54] 2012	12	Bilateral elbows, wrists, MCP2, MCP3, knees, ankles	Effusions, synovitis	Mean 22 min
Backhaus et al,[59] 2009	7	Wrist, MCP2, MCP3, PIP2, PIP3, MTP2, MTP5, all on the patient's dominant side	Erosions, synovitis, tenosynovitis	10–20 min

Abbreviations: MCP, metacarpophalangeal; MSUS, musculoskeletal ultrasound; MTP, metatarsophalangeal; PIP, proximal interphalangeal.

[a] All scoring done semiquantitatively on a scale of 0 or 1 to 3. Synovitis evaluated with combinations of gray scale and power Doppler.

patient improvement (or worsening), and often provide important prognostic information, even in the case of subclinical inflammation. Sonographic examination of all joints of the hands and feet typically involved in RA can be too time-consuming and cumbersome, and thus impractical in the clinical setting and often for research, whereas systems scoring fewer joints or views may compromise overall sensitivity too much to be useful. The proposed number of joints to scan has ranged from 78 down to 6,[53,54] although Grassi and colleagues[55] recently proposed following only "the MCP with the most florid synovitis on initial US screening," and aptly named this *one-joint* method as the SAS1 (Sonographic Activity Score) system.

Scirè and colleagues[56] used a 44-joint count scoring system to evaluate patients with early RA. Although the investigators found that MSUS was more sensitive than clinical examination in detecting disease activity, the sonographic evaluation of each patient lasted almost 1 hour. A study of patients with RA using a 28-joint count method showed similar results, with MSUS detecting more effusions and synovitis than clinical examination ($P<.05$).[13] In addition, the investigators found that a 28-joint count for effusion, synovitis, and power Doppler signal correlated well with a comprehensive 60-joint count, with the investigators stating that the 28-joint examination "can be performed in 15 minutes."

A comparative study by Dougados and colleagues,[57] who evaluated the 38-joint, 28-joint, and 20-joint MSUS synovitis scoring systems for outcome measures, found them all to be "at least as relevant as physical examination" without endorsing any particular number of joints. But they concluded that "further studies are required in order to achieve the optimal scoring system for monitoring patients…in clinical trials and in clinical practice."

On the more practical side, Perricone and colleagues[54] conducted a prospective study of 45 patients with RA starting etanercept therapy, using a 12-joint MSUS examination both at baseline and at 3-month follow-up. There was a significant correlation between changes in DAS-28 scores and changes in MSUS synovitis scores at follow-up (erosions were not reported). The same investigators then performed an analysis of a 6-joint score (bilateral wrists, second MCPs, and knees) based on the frequency of synovial abnormalities in particular locations. They found that the 6-joint score correlated significantly with baseline DAS-28 scores and was sensitive to change over a 3-month period.

Backhaus and colleagues[58,59] recently pioneered a US7 scoring system (involving the dominant wrist, second and third MCPs and proximal interphalangeal [PIP] joints, and second and fifth MTPs), which incorporates both semiquantitative grading for synovitis/tenosynovitis and the presence/absence of erosions. The investigators suggest that the 7-joint examination requires between 10 and 20 minutes to complete, and their US7 scores correlated well with DAS-28 and were sensitive to change among patients with RA on different therapeutic regimens over 1 year.

Thus, one of the current priorities of the OMERACT Ultrasound Task Force is the development of an ultrasound-based global synovitis score (GLOSS) in RA.[60] In an attempt to further clarify this issue, Mandl and colleagues[61] conducted a systematic literature review of proposed ultrasound scoring systems to establish the minimum number of joints to be included in GLOSS and analyze their metric qualities (ie, validity, reliability, feasibility). The researchers determined that, although ultrasound is a useful and powerful tool in the assessment of RA disease activity, the significant variability between studies in both defining true synovial activity and the quantitative methods used to assess synovitis made it difficult to identify the "correct" number of joints to study.

THE EMERGING ROLES OF ULTRASOUND IN RA MANAGEMENT
Solidifying Diagnoses Sooner

The ability of MSUS to detect subclinical disease and erosive changes may facilitate the ability of physicians to make an earlier diagnosis of RA and initiate treatment sooner before damage has occurred. Indeed, a 2009 study of an early arthritis cohort suggested that MSUS detected nearly 1.5 more erosions compared with radiography.[62] Moreover, a recent study by Kawashiri and colleagues[63] found that the addition of MSUS examination to the updated 2010 RA criteria in an early arthritis cohort was able to increase both sensitivity and positive predictive value of the criteria (59.5%–81.1% and 97.3%–90.0%, respectively). Similarly, a 2013 study by Nakagomi and colleagues[64] also determined that incorporation of MSUS-detected synovitis (gray-scale score ≥ 2, or power Doppler score ≥ 1) improved the specificity of the American College of Rheumatology (ACR) RA criteria (from 58.5% to 93.7%) and was better able to identify patients requiring disease-modifying anti-rheumatic drugs (DMARDs) such as methotrexate.

Assessment of Disease Activity and Treatment Response

Several studies suggest that MSUS is sensitive to treatment-related improvement. This has been shown with nonbiologic treatment with DMARDs, including a study by Naredo and colleagues[65] who demonstrated a decrease in inflammatory parameters over the course of 1 year, corroborated by MSUS, DAS-28, and radiographic progression. Numerous other studies have shown the ability of MSUS to track changes in response to biologic therapy. Iagnocco and colleagues[66] evaluated 18 patients with established RA and performed MSUS measurements before etanercept therapy and 1 year later. Using a 5-joint scoring system, the investigators found significant difference in MSUS scores between the 2 time points ($P<.0001$). A 2008 study showed similar findings using adalimumab.[67] In addition to more structured trials with anti-TNF agents, there have been a number of case series and reports of MSUS assessing disease activity in patients treated with abatacept, rituximab, and tocilizumab.[68–71]

Ultrasound as a Prognostic Tool in RA

Some studies suggest that MSUS findings can offer prognostic information to patients with RA and guide treatment changes. As mentioned in the introduction, Brown and colleagues[7] demonstrated that subclinical inflammation predicted future erosive damage. Their study also found that baseline MSUS imaging features, including (1) Doppler signal positivity, (2) synovial hypertrophy, and (3) Doppler scores, were associated with radiographic progression over 12 months in MCP joints of patients with RA, with odds ratios of 12.2, 2.3, and 4.0, respectively.

As a prognostic tool, MSUS may also be helpful in identifying which patients with RA in clinical remission are at risk for relapse (and warrant an increase in therapy). Scirè and colleagues[56] conducted a prospective study of 106 patients with RA and found that a positive power Doppler signal predicted relapse within 6 months (odds ratio 12.8, $P<.05$). A more recent study by Saleem and colleagues[72] evaluating 93 patients with RA in clinical remission concluded that both increased baseline Doppler signal and functional disability were associated with risk of relapse. Recently, an international group of rheumatologists have formed an international consortium known as the Targeted Ultrasound Initiative, to better define the role of MSUS in management of RA and to determine if more aggressive treatment of patients with subclinical sonographic synovitis alters long-term outcomes.[73]

MSUS IN JIA

JIA, the most common chronic rheumatologic disease of childhood, includes all forms of arthritis of unknown etiology presenting before the age of 16 years and lasting for at least 6 weeks. It relies heavily on physical examination to determine disease activity per the currently validated definitions,[74] although the detection of joint swelling and limited range of motion in pediatric patients varies significantly among experienced clinicians, especially in the small joints of the hand.[75]

An Evolving Diagnostic Tool

The use of MSUS in pediatric rheumatology is quickly evolving, having gained significant interest long after its application in adult rheumatology. The modality in JIA shares similar advantages with adult inflammatory diseases like RA, such as relatively low cost, dynamic images, and facility of immediate multijoint assessment. The lack of ionizing radiation, claustrophobia, or need for sedation/anesthesia with MSUS is even more appealing in the pediatric population.[76]

As in patients with RA, MSUS can demonstrate erosions, effusions, and synovial thickening in JIA.[77] Although MSUS of the knee, hands, and wrists have been studied the most in JIA,[78] sonographers can also detect intra-articular effusions and synovitis of the hips. It is more sensitive than radiographs for detecting hip joint capsule distension and early disease manifestations of JIA.[79,80] In one study, the mean distance from the femoral neck to anterior capsule ranged from 0.43 to 0.47 cm in healthy children, whereas a distance of 0.59 cm or more was found to be consistent with effusion in patients with JIA. Comparison with the contralateral hip is useful, as healthy children usually have a difference of 0.1 cm or less.[81,82]

Recent articles focusing on the evaluation of the ankle have given new insight into the complexity of ankle disease in JIA. Using MSUS as the gold standard, physical examination was insufficient to pinpoint the anatomic location of disease. Multiple compartments were affected in 80% of swollen ankles with the tibiotalar joints, subtalar joints, midfoot joints, and tendons involved.[83,84] Isolated tibiotalar disease occurred in less than 30% of swollen ankles, whereas tenosynovitis was a common finding and more likely to affect the medial tendons in patients with oligoarthritis.

Because synovial hypertrophy may persist in clinically inactive disease, Doppler ultrasound may be useful to detect inflammatory blood flow, and has also been used to monitor response to therapy in JIA.[85,86] Conventional inflammatory markers may be normal in juvenile arthritis, and power Doppler is more sensitive than ESR and CRP to detect active disease.[87] Entheseal inflammation detected by power Doppler ultrasound is an infrequent finding in patients with nonenthesitis-related JIA. Power Doppler signal–detected enthesitis occurs in less than 10% of patients with oligoarticular and polyarticular arthritis. The presence of power Doppler correlates with clinical enthesitis, bursitis, and erosions, but not with tendon thickening.[88]

The use of MSUS for targeted corticosteroid injections in JIA is safe and effective.[84,89–91] Ultrasound can be used to guide injections of small, medium, and large joints and tendon sheaths. Complications appear to be infrequent, but include subcutaneous atrophy, skin hypopigmentation, erythema, and pruritus. Despite the paucity of evidence supporting its use for diagnosis of temporomandibular joint (TMJ) arthritis,[92,93] MSUS has been used to guide injections of the TMJ in children with arthritis with accurate placement confirmed by computed tomography in 91% of cases.[94,95]

Limitations and Lack of Validated Scoring Systems

In contrast to MSUS in RA, currently there are no specific definitions for ultrasonographic pathology in children with JIA. It is unclear if definitions of bone erosion, synovial effusion, synovial hypertrophy, tenosynovitis, and enthesopathy described in the adult literature are directly applicable to children,[30] as knowledge of normal sonographic findings unique to the growing child is critical to avoid misinterpretation. For example, vascularization may be present in cartilage and tendons of healthy children,[96] and cartilage thickness decreases as children grow and varies between sexes.[97] Doppler signal can look similar in hypertrophic synovitis and healthy cartilaginous epiphyses during growth, thus careful anatomic assessment is required to differentiate which well-vascularized tissue is being viewed.[98] Bony ossification may appear wavy, irregular, and fragmented (**Fig. 4**), and careful interpretation is required to avoid an inaccurate diagnosis of erosions or enthesitis from JIA.

In addition, there are discrepancies between the clinical examination and MSUS findings of patients with JIA.[99–104] MSUS has often failed to confirm synovitis in joints determined to be abnormal by physical examination. Conversely, it also detects subclinical synovitis in some asymptomatic joints (specifically the hands and feet) in active

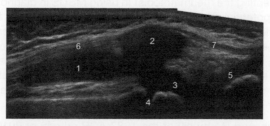

Fig. 4. An 18-month-old patient with JIA, anterior longitudinal view of the knee. Note (1) suprapatellar recess distended by effusion and synovial hypertrophy, (2) unossified patella, (3) unossified distal femoral epiphysis, (4) distal femoral physis, (5) proximal tibial epiphysis, (6) quadriceps tendon, and (7) patellar tendon.

patients, and has also demonstrated synovial abnormalities in patients with clinically inactive disease. Rebollo-Pollo and colleagues[105] suggest that this finding may indicate persistent inflammation, whereas another longitudinal study found that ultrasound-detected synovial abnormalities were not predictive of flare.[106] These findings could affect treatment decisions, as the detection of subclinical synovitis could result in reclassification of the patient from the oligoarthritis to polyarthritis subtype of JIA.[107]

There are sparse data comparing MSUS with other imaging modalities for the detection of erosions in JIA. Malattia and colleagues[108] found that MRI detected more erosions than MSUS or plain radiography in assessing the wrists, which may not be surprising given the complexity of the pediatric wrist joint. Another study found similar results when comparing MRI with MSUS but did not focus on a specific joint and compared only a small number of patients.[109] In a noncomparative study, Karmazyn and colleagues[110] found that erosions of MCP joints of patients with JIA can be detected with MSUS. The observed location of erosions varies by age, with marginal erosions occurring in the teenager, and epiphyseal erosions more common at a younger age (average of 8.7 years). Additional studies are needed to clearly define the role of MSUS to detect erosions in children.

Recent literature consistently encourage the pediatric rheumatologist to proceed in using MSUS with patients with JIA, but do so with caution given the complex (sono) anatomy of the growing child and the current lack of any validated ultrasound scoring systems or treatment algorithms.[98]

PROPOSED ALGORITHMS USING MSUS IN RA

The ACR recently released a report on "reasonable use" of MSUS in clinical practice, suggesting 14 different clinical scenarios in which it would be helpful and appropriate to scan specific joints.[111] Although the Committee used the RAND/University of California Los Angeles method to compile its recommendations for all aspects of MSUS use in rheumatology (without specific mention of RA), it addressed the "uncertainty and focus of [the] literature" advocating MSUS. The report's only scenario applicable to supporting MSUS in the diagnosis or management of RA referred to "inflammatory arthritis" in general, not commenting on the frequency or anatomic breadth of the examinations: "For a patient with diagnosed inflammatory arthritis and new or ongoing symptoms without definitive diagnosis on clinical examination, it is reasonable to use MSUS to evaluate for inflammatory disease activity, structural damage, or emergence of an alternate cause" at a variety of anatomic sites.

With this report mind, as well as the lack of any other concise evidence-based recommendations directing the rheumatologist in using MSUS in diagnosing and managing RA, we offer 3 potential clinical scenarios with recommendations for diagnosis and assessment of sonographic disease activity. A patient's outcome from these scenario options can then be applied to the ACR's recently revised RA treatment recommendations using MSUS data (erosions, effusions, and synovitis) in place of plain radiography erosions to assess the patient and progress through the treatment algorithms with respect to use of DMARDs and biologics. Here are the 3 scenarios and our recommendations for each:

1. Previously diagnosed RA by either the 1987 ACR criteria or 2010 ACR-European League Against Rheumatism (EULAR) Classification criteria, with active disease:
   a. Perform the US7 and also scan any other active or painful joint by gray scale and Doppler for baseline data.

   b. Reimage 3 months after any DMARD/biologic change to document any change in synovitis or emergence or any new erosions.

   c. Once the patient is stable clinically and sonographically on the same regimen for at least 3 months, reimage annually to rule out ongoing subclinical damage.

2. Previously diagnosed RA by either the 1987 ACR criteria or 2010 ACR-EULAR Classification criteria, but currently quiescent without synovitis:

   a. Perform the US7 for baseline data.

   b. Reimage annually to rule out ongoing subclinical damage, or sooner if there is any worsening of symptoms.

   c. Reimage 3 months after any DMARD/biologic change.

3. Undiagnosed seronegative inflammatory polyarthritis for more than 6 weeks, and RA is under consideration:

   a. Perform the US7 and also scan any other active or painful joint by gray scale and Doppler for baseline data.

   b. Scan carefully to exclude gout, chondrocalcinosis, enthesitis, or infections/diseases that might mimic RA clinically. Reimage 3 months after any DMARD/biologic change to document any change in synovitis or emergence or any new erosions.

   c. Once the patient is stable clinically and sonographically on the same regimen for at least 3 months, reimage annually to rule out ongoing subclinical damage.

We also suggest that in unexplained polyarthritis or in previously diagnosed RA in which the clinical picture makes the diagnosis questionable, MSUS images should be given consideration to reassess the diagnosis. For example, one reported case of bilateral MCP polyarthritis revealed subcutaneous nodules but no intra-articular fluid or synovitis, leading to the proper diagnosis of an Infection with *Mycobacterium marinum*.[112] Overall, it is important to state that the MSUS findings need to be placed into the context of the rest of the patient's clinical picture, and that physicians not treat based on MSUS findings alone.

SUMMARY

The management of RA and JIA has increasingly incorporated the use of MSUS to provide diagnostic and prognostic information and assess patients' responses to therapy, especially with regard to erosions, effusions, synovitis, and tenosynovitis. The modality allows physicians to view important anatomic structures more quickly, dynamically, and with fewer complications and contraindications than other imaging modalities, providing important information about disease activity and damage that is not available by physical examination or plain radiography. Indeed, the ability of both clinician and patient to simultaneously visualize pathology can reassure both of them, and help them to make rational treatment decisions together.

At this time, we have many proposed scoring systems but lack a universally accepted method or number of required joints to study for either RA or JIA, likely hampering the incorporation of MSUS into accepted treatment algorithms or remission criteria in either disease. This limitation is more apparent in JIA, as the complexity of imaging the child's developing anatomy has made the validation of a scoring system even more challenging. Still, it is imperative for rheumatologists to further develop expertise using this modality in clinical practice, and spur the creation of well-designed studies that incorporate ultrasound into current diagnostic and remission criteria. As investigators refine reliable scoring systems in both RA and JIA, it may become easier to incorporate MSUS into the diseases' treatment algorithms and further solidify its role in routine management and in the future of rheumatology.

REFERENCES

1. Aretha D, Neoga T, Salman AJ, et al. 2010 Rheumatoid arthritis classification criteria: an American College of Rheumatology/European League Against Rheumatism collaborative initiative. Arthritis Rheum 2010;62:2569–81.
2. Machine H, Kautiainen H, Hannonen P, et al. Is DAS28 an appropriate tool to assess remission in rheumatoid arthritis? Ann Rheum Dis 2005;64:1410–3.
3. Wolfe F, Michaud K, Pincus T, et al. The disease activity score is not suitable as the sole criterion for initiation and evaluation of anti-tumor necrosis factor therapy in the clinic: discordance between assessment measures and limitations in questionnaire use for regulatory purposes. Arthritis Rheum 2005;52: 3873–9.
4. Keenan RT, Swearingen CJ, Yazici Y. Erythrocyte sedimentation rate and C-reactive protein levels are poorly correlated with clinical measures of disease activity in rheumatoid arthritis, systemic lupus erythematosus and osteoarthritis patients. Clin Exp Rheumatol 2008;26:814–9.
5. Matsui T, Kuga Y, Kaneko A, et al. Disease Activity Score 28 (DAS28) using C-reactive protein underestimates disease activity and overestimates EULAR response criteria compared with DAS28 using erythrocyte sedimentation rate in a large observational cohort of rheumatoid arthritis patients in Japan. Ann Rheum Dis 2007;66:1221–6.
6. D'Agostino MA, Breban M. Ultrasonography in inflammatory joint disease: why should rheumatologists pay attention? Joint Bone Spine 2002;69:252–5.
7. Brown AK, Conaghan PG, Karim Z, et al. An explanation for the apparent dissociation between clinical remission and continued structural deterioration in rheumatoid arthritis. Arthritis Rheum 2008;58:2958–67.
8. McDonald D, Leopold G. Ultrasound B-scanning in the differentiation of Baker's cyst and thrombophlebitis. Br J Radiol 1972;45:729–32.
9. Cooperberg PL, Tsang I, Truelove L, et al. Gray scale ultrasound in the evaluation of rheumatoid arthritis of the knee. Radiology 1978;126:759–63.
10. Grassi W, Tittarelli E, Pirani O, et al. Ultrasound examination of metacarpophalangeal joints in rheumatoid arthritis. Scand J Rheumatol 1993;22:243–7.
11. Lund PJ, Heikal A, Maricic MJ, et al. Ultrasonographic imaging of the hand and wrist in rheumatoid arthritis. Skeletal Radiol 1995;24:591–6.
12. Backhaus M, Kamradt T, Sandrock D, et al. Arthritis of the finger joints: a comprehensive approach comparing conventional radiography, scintigraphy, ultrasound, and contrast-enhanced magnetic resonance imaging. Arthritis Rheum 1999;42:1232–45.
13. Naredo E, Bonilla G, Gamero F, et al. Assessment of inflammatory activity in rheumatoid arthritis: a comparative study of clinical evaluation with grey scale and power Doppler ultrasonography. Ann Rheum Dis 2005;64:375–81.
14. Szkudlarek M, Klarlund M, Narvestad E, et al. Ultrasonography of the metacarpophalangeal and proximal interphalangeal joints in rheumatoid arthritis: a comparison with magnetic resonance imaging, conventional radiography and clinical examination. Arthritis Res Ther 2006;8:R52.
15. Wakefield RJ, Freeston JE, O'Connor P, et al. The optimal assessment of the rheumatoid arthritis hindfoot: a comparative study of clinical examination, ultrasound and high field MRI. Ann Rheum Dis 2008;67:1678–82.
16. Rahmani M, Chegini H, Najafizadeh SR, et al. Detection of bone erosion in early rheumatoid arthritis: ultrasonography and conventional radiography versus non-contrast magnetic resonance imaging. Clin Rheumatol 2010;29:883–91.

17. Freeston JE, Brown AK, Hensor EM, et al. Extremity magnetic resonance imaging assessment of synovitis (without contrast) in rheumatoid arthritis may be less accurate than power Doppler ultrasound. Ann Rheum Dis 2008;67:1351.

18. Foltz V, Gandjbakhch F, Etchepare F, et al. Power Doppler ultrasound, but not low-field magnetic resonance imaging, predicts relapse and radiographic disease progression in rheumatoid arthritis patients with low levels of disease activity. Arthritis Rheum 2012;64:67–76.

19. Swen WA, Jacobs JW, Hubach PC, et al. Comparison of sonography and magnetic resonance imaging for the diagnosis of partial tears of finger extensor tendons in rheumatoid arthritis. Rheumatology 2000;39:55–62.

20. Wakefield RJ, Balint PV, Szkudlarek M, et al. Musculoskeletal ultrasound including definitions for ultrasonographic pathology. J Rheumatol 2005;32: 2485–7.

21. Wakefield RJ, D'Agostino MA, Iagnocco A, et al. The OMERACT Ultrasound Group: status of current activities and research directions. J Rheumatol 2007; 34:848–51.

22. Brown AK. Using ultrasonography to facilitate best practice in diagnosis and management of RA. Nat Rev Rheumatol 2009;5:698–706.

23. Jain M, Samuels J. Musculoskeletal ultrasound as a diagnostic and prognostic tool in rheumatoid arthritis. Bull NYU Hosp Jt Dis 2011;69:215–9.

24. Boutry N, Morel M, Flipo RM, et al. Early rheumatoid arthritis: a review of MRI and sonographic findings. Am J Roentgenol 2007;189:1502–9.

25. Wakefield RJ, Gibbon WW, Conaghan PG, et al. The value of sonography in the detection of bone erosions in patients with rheumatoid arthritis: a comparison with conventional radiography. Arthritis Rheum 2000;43:2762–70.

26. Lopez-Ben R, Bernreuter WK, Moreland LW, et al. Ultrasound detection of bone erosions in rheumatoid arthritis: a comparison to routine radiographs of the hands and feet. Skeletal Radiol 2004;32:80–4.

27. Ostergaard M, Szkudlarek M. Imaging in rheumatoid arthritis—why MRI and ultrasonography can no longer be ignored. Scand J Rheumatol 2003;32:63–73.

28. Szkudlarek M, Court-Payen M, Jacobsen S, et al. Interobserver agreement in ultrasonography of the finger and toe joints in rheumatoid arthritis. Arthritis Rheum 2003;48:955–62.

29. Gutierrez M, Filippucci E, Ruta S, et al. Inter-observer reliability of high-resolution ultrasonography in the assessment of bone erosions in patients with rheumatoid arthritis: experience of an intensive dedicated training programme. Rheumatology 2011;50:373–80.

30. Wakefield RJ, Balint PV, Szkudlarek M, et al, OMERACT 7 Special Interest Group. Musculoskeletal ultrasound including definitions for ultrasonographic pathology. J Rheumatol 2005;32:2485–7.

31. Tan YK, Conaghan P. Imaging in rheumatoid arthritis. Best Pract Res Clin Rheumatol 2011;25:569–84.

32. Walther M, Harms H, Krenn V, et al. Correlation of power Doppler sonography with vascularity of the synovial tissue of the knee joint in patients with osteoarthritis and rheumatoid arthritis. Arthritis Rheum 2001;44:331–8.

33. Walther M, Harms H, Krenn V, et al. Synovial tissue of the hip at power Doppler US: correlation between vascularity and power Doppler US signal. Radiology 2002;225:225–31.

34. Boutry N, Lardé A, Lapègue F, et al. Magnetic resonance imaging appearance of the hands and feet in patients with early rheumatoid arthritis. J Rheumatol 2003;30:671–9.

35. Micu MC, Serra S, Fodor D, et al. Inter-observer reliability of ultrasound detection of tendon abnormalities at the wrist and ankle in patients with rheumatoid arthritis. Rheumatology 2011;50:1120–4.
36. Bruyn GA, Möller I, Garrido J, et al. Reliability testing of tendon disease using two different scanning methods in patients with rheumatoid arthritis. Rheumatology 2012;51:1655–61.
37. Weiner SM, Jurenz S, Uhl M, et al. Ultrasonography in the assessment of peripheral joint involvement in psoriatic arthritis: a comparison with radiography, MRI and scintigraphy. Clin Rheumatol 2008;27:983–9.
38. Balint PV, Kane D, Wilson H, et al. Ultrasonography of entheseal insertions in the lower limb in spondyloarthropathy. Ann Rheum Dis 2002;61:905–10.
39. Freeston JE, Coates LC, Helliwell PS, et al. Is there subclinical enthesitis in early psoriatic arthritis? A clinical comparison with power Doppler ultrasound. Arthritis Care Res 2012;64:1617–21.
40. Gutierrez M, Di Geso L, Salaffi F, et al. Development of a preliminary US power Doppler composite score for monitoring treatment in PsA. Rheumatology 2012; 51:1261–8.
41. Wiell C, Szkudlarek M, Hasselquist M, et al. Ultrasonography, magnetic resonance imaging, radiography, and clinical assessment of inflammatory and destructive changes in fingers and toes of patients with psoriatic arthritis. Arthritis Res Ther 2007;9:R119.
42. Teoli M, Zangrilli A, Chimenti MS, et al. Evaluation of clinical and ultrasonographic parameters in psoriatic arthritis patients treated with adalimumab: a retrospective study. Clin Dev Immunol 2012;2012:823854.
43. Thiele RG, Schlesinger N. Diagnosis of gout by ultrasound. Rheumatology 2007; 46:1116–21.
44. Filippucci E, Riveros MG, Georgescu D, et al. Hyaline cartilage involvement in patients with gout and calcium pyrophosphate deposition disease. An ultrasound study. Osteoarthr Cartil 2009;17:178–81.
45. Ottaviani S, Richette P, Allard A, et al. Ultrasonography in gout: a case-control study. Clin Exp Rheumatol 2012;30:499–504.
46. Thiele RG, Schlesinger N. Ultrasonography shows disappearance of monosodium urate crystal deposition on hyaline cartilage after sustained normouricemia is achieved. Rheumatol Int 2010;30:495–503.
47. Nalbant S, Corominas H, Hsu B, et al. Ultrasonography for assessment of subcutaneous nodules. J Rheumatol 2003;30:1191–5.
48. de Ávila Fernandes E, Kubota ES, Sandim GB, et al. Ultrasound features of tophi in chronic tophaceous gout. Skeletal Radiol 2011;40:309–15.
49. Wright SA, Filippucci E, McVeigh C, et al. High-resolution ultrasonography of the first metatarsal phalangeal joint in gout: a controlled study. Ann Rheum Dis 2007;66:859–64.
50. Howard RG, Pillinger MH, Gyftopoulos S, et al. Reproducibility of musculoskeletal ultrasound for determining monosodium urate deposition: concordance between readers. Arthritis Care Res 2011;63:1456–62.
51. Frediani B, Filippou G, Falsetti P, et al. Diagnosis of calcium pyrophosphate dihydrate crystal deposition disease: ultrasonographic criteria proposed. Ann Rheum Dis 2005;64:638–40.
52. Conaghan PG, D'Agostino MA, Le Bars M, et al. Clinical and ultrasonographic predictors of joint replacement for knee osteoarthritis: results from a large, 3-year, prospective EULAR study. Ann Rheum Dis 2010;69:644–7.

53. Hammer HB, Sveinsson M, Kongtorp AK, et al. A 78-joints ultrasonographic assessment is associated with clinical assessments and is highly responsive to improvement in a longitudinal study of patients with rheumatoid arthritis starting adalimumab treatment. Ann Rheum Dis 2010;69:1349–51.

54. Perricone C, Ceccarelli F, Modesti M, et al. The 6-joint ultrasonographic assessment: a valid, sensitive-to-change and feasible method for evaluating joint inflammation in RA. Rheumatology 2012;51:866–73.

55. Grassi W, Gaywood I, Pande I, et al. From DAS 28 to SAS 1. Clin Exp Rheumatol 2012;30:649–51.

56. Scirè CA, Montecucco C, Codullo V, et al. Ultrasonographic evaluation of joint involvement in early rheumatoid arthritis in clinical remission: power Doppler signal predicts short-term relapse. Rheumatology 2009;48:1092–7.

57. Dougados M, Jousse-Joulin S, Mistretta F, et al. Evaluation of several ultrasonography scoring systems for synovitis and comparison to clinical examination: results from a prospective multicentre study of rheumatoid arthritis. Ann Rheum Dis 2010;69:828–33.

58. Backhaus TM, Ohrndorf S, Kellner H, et al. The US7 score is sensitive to change in a large cohort of patients with rheumatoid arthritis over 12 months of therapy. Ann Rheum Dis 2012. [Epub ahead of print].

59. Backhaus M, Ohrndorf S, Kellner H, et al. Evaluation of a novel 7-joint ultrasound score in daily rheumatologic practice: a pilot project. Arthritis Rheum 2009;61: 1194–201.

60. Naredo E, Wakefield RJ, Iagnocco A, et al. The OMERACT ultrasound task force—status and perspectives. J Rheumatol 2011;38:2063–7.

61. Mandl P, Naredo E, Wakefield RJ, et al, OMERACT Ultrasound Task Force. A systematic literature review analysis of ultrasound joint count and scoring systems to assess synovitis in rheumatoid arthritis according to the OMERACT filter. J Rheumatol 2011;38:2055–62.

62. Funck-Brentano T, Etchepare F, Joulin SJ, et al. Benefits of ultrasonography in the management of early arthritis: a cross-sectional study of baseline data from the ESPOIR cohort. Rheumatology 2009;48:1515–9.

63. Kawashiri SY, Suzuki T, Okada A, et al. Musculoskeletal ultrasonography assists the diagnostic performance of the 2010 classification criteria for rheumatoid arthritis. Mod Rheumatol 2012;23:36–43.

64. Nakagomi D, Ikeda K, Okubo A, et al. Ultrasound can improve the accuracy of the 2010 ACR/EULAR classification criteria for rheumatoid arthritis to predict methotrexate requirement. Arthritis Rheum 2013. http://dx.doi.org/10.1002/art.37848.

65. Naredo E, Collado P, Cruz A, et al. Longitudinal power Doppler ultrasonographic assessment of joint inflammatory activity in early rheumatoid arthritis: predictive value in disease activity and radiologic progression. Arthritis Rheum 2007;57: 116–24.

66. Iagnocco A, Perella C, Naredo E, et al. Etanercept in the treatment of rheumatoid arthritis: clinical follow-up over one year by ultrasonography. Clin Rheumatol 2008;27:491–6.

67. Iagnocco A, Filippucci E, Perella C, et al. Clinical and ultrasonographic monitoring of response to adalimumab treatment in rheumatoid arthritis. J Rheumatol 2008; 35:35–40.

68. Kawashiri SY, Fujikawa K, Nishino A, et al. Usefulness of ultrasonography-proven tenosynovitis to monitor disease activity of a patient with very early

rheumatoid arthritis treated by abatacept. Mod Rheumatol 2012. [Epub ahead of print].

69. Epis O, Filippucci E, Delle Sedie A, et al. Clinical and ultrasound evaluation of the response to tocilizumab treatment in patients with rheumatoid arthritis: a case series. Rheumatol Int 2013. [Epub ahead of print].

70. Hama M, Uehara T, Takase K, et al. Power Doppler ultrasonography is useful for assessing disease activity and predicting joint destruction in rheumatoid arthritis patients receiving tocilizumab—preliminary data. Rheumatol Int 2012; 32:1327–33.

71. Ziswiler HR, Aeberli D, Villiger PM, et al. High-resolution ultrasound confirms reduced synovial hyperplasia following rituximab treatment in rheumatoid arthritis. Rheumatology (Oxford) 2009;48:939–43.

72. Saleem B, Brown AK, Quinn M, et al. Can flare be predicted in DMARD treated RA patients in remission, and is it important? A cohort study. Ann Rheum Dis 2012;71:1316–21.

73. Wakefield RJ, D'Agostino MA, Naredo E, et al. After treat-to-target: can a targeted ultrasound initiative improve RA outcomes? Ann Rheum Dis 2012;71:799–803.

74. Wallace CA, Ruperto N, Giannini E. Preliminary criteria for clinical remission for select categories of juvenile idiopathic arthritis. J Rheumatol 2004;31:2290–4.

75. Guzman J, Burgos-Vargas R, Duarte-Salazar C, et al. Reliability of the articular examination in children with juvenile rheumatoid arthritis: interobserver agreement and sources of disagreement. J Rheumatol 1995;22:2331–6.

76. Damasio MB, Malattia C, Martini A, et al. Synovial and inflammatory diseases in childhood: role of new imaging modalities in the assessment of patients with juvenile idiopathic arthritis. Pediatr Radiol 2010;40:985–98.

77. Cellerini M, Salti S, Trapani S, et al. Correlation between clinical and ultrasound assessment of the knee in children with mono-articular or pauci-articular juvenile rheumatoid arthritis. Pediatr Radiol 1999;29:117–23.

78. Collado P, Jousse-Joulin S, Alcalde M, et al. Is ultrasound a validated imaging tool for the diagnosis and management of synovitis in juvenile idiopathic arthritis? A systematic literature review. Arthritis Care Res 2012;64:1011–9.

79. Fedrizzi MS, Ronchezel MV, Hilario MO, et al. Ultrasonography in the early diagnosis of hip joint involvement in juvenile rheumatoid arthritis. J Rheumatol 1997; 24:1820–5.

80. Martinoli C, Garello I, Marchetti A, et al. Hip ultrasound. Eur J Radiol 2012;81: 3824–31.

81. Robben SG, Lequin MH, Diepstraten AF, et al. Anterior joint capsule of the normal hip and in children with transient synovitis: US study with anatomic and histologic correlation. Radiology 1999;210:499–507.

82. Friedman S, Gruber MA. Ultrasonography of the hip in the evaluation of children with seronegative juvenile rheumatoid arthritis. J Rheumatol 2002;29:629–32.

83. Pascoli L, Wright S, McAllister C, et al. Prospective evaluation of clinical and ultrasound findings in ankle disease in juvenile idiopathic arthritis: importance of ankle ultrasound. J Rheumatol 2010;37:2409–14.

84. Laurell L, Court-Payen M, Nielsen S, et al. Ultrasonography and color Doppler in juvenile idiopathic arthritis: diagnosis and follow-up of ultrasound-guided steroid injection in the ankle region. A descriptive interventional study. Pediatr Rheumatol Online J 2011;9:4.

85. Shanmugavel C, Sodhi KS, Sandhu MS, et al. Role of power Doppler sonography in evaluation of therapeutic response of the knee in juvenile rheumatoid arthritis. Rheumatol Int 2008;28:573–8.

86. Shahin AA, el-Mofty SA, el-Sheikh EA, et al. Power Doppler sonography in the evaluation and follow-up of knee involvement in patients with juvenile idiopathic arthritis. Z Rheumatol 2001;60:148–55.

87. Sparchez M, Fodor D, Miu N. The role of power Doppler ultrasonography in comparison with biological markers in the evaluation of disease activity in juvenile idiopathic arthritis. Med Ultrason 2010;12:97–103.

88. Jousse-Joulin S, Breton S, Cangemi C, et al. Ultrasonography for detecting enthesitis in juvenile idiopathic arthritis. Arthritis Care Res 2011;63:849–55.

89. Young CM, Shiels WE 2nd, Coley BD, et al. Ultrasound-guided corticosteroid injection therapy for juvenile idiopathic arthritis: 12-year care experience. Pediatr Radiol 2012;42:1481–9.

90. Laurell L, Court-Payen M, Nielsen S, et al. Ultrasonography and color Doppler in juvenile idiopathic arthritis: diagnosis and follow-up of ultrasound-guided steroid injection in the wrist region. A descriptive interventional study. Pediatr Rheumatol Online J 2012;10:11.

91. Tynjala P, Honkanen V, Lahdenne P. Intra-articular steroids in radiologically confirmed tarsal and hip synovitis of juvenile idiopathic arthritis. Clin Exp Rheumatol 2004;22:643–8.

92. Weiss PF, Arabshahi B, Johnson A, et al. High prevalence of temporomandibular joint arthritis at disease onset in children with juvenile idiopathic arthritis, as detected by magnetic resonance imaging but not by ultrasound. Arthritis Rheum 2008;58:1189–96.

93. Muller L, Kellenberger CJ, Cannizzaro E, et al. Early diagnosis of temporomandibular joint involvement in juvenile idiopathic arthritis: a pilot study comparing clinical examination and ultrasound to magnetic resonance imaging. Rheumatology (Oxford) 2009;48:680–5.

94. Habibi S, Ellis J, Strike H, et al. Safety and efficacy of US-guided CS injection into temporomandibular joints in children with active JIA. Rheumatology (Oxford) 2012;51:874–7.

95. Parra DA, Chan M, Krishnamurthy G, et al. Use and accuracy of US guidance for image-guided injections of the temporomandibular joints in children with arthritis. Pediatr Radiol 2010;40:1498–504.

96. Grechenig W, Mayr JM, Peicha G, et al. Sonoanatomy of the Achilles tendon insertion in children. J Clin Ultrasound 2004;32:338–43.

97. Spannow AH, Pfeiffer-Jensen M, Andersen NT, et al. Ultrasonographic measurements of joint cartilage thickness in healthy children: age- and sex-related standard reference values. J Rheumatol 2010;37:2595–601.

98. Laurell L, Court-Payen M, Boesen M, et al. Imaging in juvenile idiopathic arthritis with a focus on ultrasonography. Clin Exp Rheumatol 2013;31:135–48.

99. Magni-Manzoni S, Epis O, Ravelli A, et al. Comparison of clinical versus ultrasound-determined synovitis in juvenile idiopathic arthritis. Arthritis Rheum 2009;61:1497–504.

100. Haslam KE, McCann LJ, Wyatt S, et al. The detection of subclinical synovitis by ultrasound in oligoarticular juvenile idiopathic arthritis: a pilot study. Rheumatology (Oxford) 2010;49:123–7.

101. Filippou G, Cantarini L, Bertoldi I, et al. Ultrasonography vs. clinical examination in children with suspected arthritis. Does it make sense to use poliarticular ultrasonographic screening? Clin Exp Rheumatol 2011;29:345–50.

102. Hendry GJ, Gardner-Medwin J, Steultjens MP, et al. Frequent discordance between clinical and musculoskeletal ultrasound examinations of foot disease in juvenile idiopathic arthritis. Arthritis Care Res 2012;64:441–7.

103. Breton S, Jousse-Joulin S, Cangemi C, et al. Comparison of clinical and ultrasonographic evaluations for peripheral synovitis in juvenile idiopathic arthritis. Semin Arthritis Rheum 2011;41:272-8.

104. Janow GL, Panghaal V, Trinh A, et al. Detection of active disease in juvenile idiopathic arthritis: sensitivity and specificity of the physical examination vs ultrasound. J Rheumatol 2011;38:2671-4.

105. Rebollo-Polo M, Koujok K, Weisser C, et al. Ultrasound findings on patients with juvenile idiopathic arthritis in clinical remission. Arthritis Care Res 2011;63: 1013-9.

106. Magni-Manzoni S, Scire CA, Ravelli A, et al. Ultrasound-detected synovial abnormalities are frequent in clinically inactive juvenile idiopathic arthritis, but do not predict a flare of synovitis. Ann Rheum Dis 2013;72:223-8.

107. Petty RE, Southwood TR, Manners P, et al. International League of Associations for Rheumatology classification of juvenile idiopathic arthritis: second revision, Edmonton, 2001. J Rheumatol 2004;31:390-2.

108. Malattia C, Damasio MB, Magnaguagno F, et al. Magnetic resonance imaging, ultrasonography, and conventional radiography in the assessment of bone erosions in juvenile idiopathic arthritis. Arthritis Rheum 2008;59:1764-72.

109. Laurell L, Court-Payen M, Nielsen S, et al. Comparison of ultrasonography with Doppler and MRI for assessment of disease activity in juvenile idiopathic arthritis: a pilot study. Pediatr Rheumatol Online J 2012;10:23.

110. Karmazyn B, Bowyer SL, Schmidt KM, et al. US findings of metacarpophalangeal joints in children with idiopathic juvenile arthritis. Pediatr Radiol 2007;37: 475-82.

111. McAlindon T, Kissin E, Nazarian L, et al. American College of Rheumatology report on reasonable use of musculoskeletal ultrasonography in rheumatology clinical practice. Arthritis Care Res 2012;64:1625-40.

112. Furer V, Franks AG, Magro CM, et al. Musculoskeletal ultrasound prompts a rare diagnosis of Mycobacterium marinum infection. Scand J Rheumatol 2012;41: 316-8.

113. Alarcon GS, Lopez-Ben R, Moreland LW. High-resolution ultrasound for the study of target joints in rheumatoid arthritis. Arthritis Rheum 2002;46:1969-70 [author reply: 70-1].

114. Abraham AM, Goff I, Pearce MS, et al. Reliability and validity of ultrasound imaging of features of knee osteoarthritis in the community. BMC Musculoskelet Disord 2011;12:70.

Index

Note: Page numbers of article titles are in **boldface** type.

A

B

Rheum Dis Clin N Am 39 (2013) 689–699
http://dx.doi.org/10.1016/S0889-857X(13)00057-4   **rheumatic.theclinics.com**
0889-857X/13/$ – see front matter © 2013 Elsevier Inc. All rights reserved.

Printed and bound by CPI Group (UK) Ltd, Croydon, CR0 4YY

03/10/2024

01040442-0016